普通高等教育中医药类"十三五"规划教材

全国普通高等教育中医药类精编教材

中 医 英 语

（第 3 版）

（供中医学、针灸推拿学、中西医临床医学等专业用）

U0188405

主　编

施建蓉　周　恩

副主编

（按姓氏拼音排序）

陈　骥　董敏华　范延妮　郭先英

李涛安　李晓莉　刘　娅　徐永红

国际主审

Sean Bradley

国内主审

丁年青

本书配套数字教学资源

微信扫描二维码，加入中医英语读者交流圈，获取配套教学视频、学习课件、课后习题和沟通交流平台等板块内容，夯实基础知识

上海科学技术出版社

图书在版编目（CIP）数据

中医英语 / 施建蓉，周恩主编. -- 3版. -- 上海 ：
上海科学技术出版社，2020.8（2025.1重印）
普通高等教育中医药类"十三五"规划教材　全国普
通高等教育中医药类精编教材
ISBN 978-7-5478-4970-5

Ⅰ．①中… Ⅱ．①施… ②周… Ⅲ．①中国医药学－
英语－中医学院－教材 Ⅳ．①R2

中国版本图书馆CIP数据核字(2020)第104361号

中医英语(第3版)

主编　施建蓉　周　恩

上海世纪出版(集团)有限公司
上 海 科 学 技 术 出 版 社　出版、发行
(上海市闵行区号景路 159 弄 A 座 9F - 10F)
邮政编码 201101　www.sstp.cn
浙江新华印刷技术有限公司印刷
开本 787×1092　1/16　印张 15.25
字数 380 千字
2009 年 8 月第 1 版
2020 年 8 月第 3 版　2025 年 1 月第 23 次印刷
ISBN 978 - 7 - 5478 - 4970 - 5/R · 2113
定价：45.00 元

普通高等教育中医药类"十三五"规划教材
全国普通高等教育中医药类精编教材

普通高等教育中医药类"十三五"规划教材
全国普通高等教育中医药类精编教材

前　言

新中国高等中医药教育开创至今历六十年。一甲子朝花夕拾，六十年砥砺前行，实现了长足发展，不仅健全了中医药高等教育体系，创新了中医药高等教育模式，也培养了一大批中医药人才，履行了人才培养、科技创新、社会服务、文化传承的职能和使命。高等中医药院校的教材作为中医药知识传播的重要载体，也伴随着中医药高等教育改革发展的进程，从少到多，从粗到精，一纲多本，形式多样，始终发挥着至关重要的作用。

上海科学技术出版社于1964年受国家卫生部委托出版全国中医院校试用教材迄今，肩负了半个多世纪的中医院校教材建设和出版的重任，产生了一大批学术深厚、内涵丰富、文辞隽永、具有重要影响力的优秀教材。尤其是1985年出版的全国统编高等医学院校中医教材(第五版)，至今仍被誉为中医教材之经典而蜚声海内外。

2006年，上海科学技术出版社在全国中医药高等教育学会教学管理研究会的精心指导下，在全国各中医药院校的积极参与下，组织出版了供中医药院校本科生使用的"全国普通高等教育中医药类精编教材"(以下简称"精编教材")，并于2011年进行了修订和完善。这套教材融汇了历版优秀教材之精华，遵循"三基""五性""三特定"的教材编写原则，同时高度契合国家执业医师考核制度改革和国家创新型人才培养战略的要求，在组织策划、编写和出版过程中，反复论证，层层把关，使"精编教材"在内容编写、版式设计和质量控制等方面均达到了预期的要求，凸显了"精炼、创新、适用"的编写初衷，获得了全国中医药院校师生的一致好评。

2016年8月，党中央、国务院召开了新世纪以来第一次全国卫生与健康大会，印发实施《"健康中国2030"规划纲要》，并颁布了《中医药法》和《〈中国的中医药〉白皮书》，把发展中医药事业作为打造健康中国的重要内容。实施创新驱动发展、文化强国、"走出去"战略以及"一带一路"倡议，推动经济转型升级，都需要中医药发挥资源优势和核心作用。面对新时期中医药"创造性转化，创新性发展"的总体要求，中医药高等教育必须牢牢把握经济社会发展的大势，更加主动地服务和融入国家发展战略。为此，精编教材的编写将继续秉持"为院校提供服务、为行业打造精品"的工作要旨，在全国中医院校中广泛征求意见,多方听取要求,全面汲取经验,经过近一年的精心准备工作,在"十三五"开局之年启动了第三版的修订工作。

本次修订和完善将在保持"精编教材"原有特色和优势的基础上,进一步突出"经典、精炼、新颖、实用"的特点,并将贯彻习近平总书记在全国卫生与健康大会、全国高校思想政治工作会议等系列讲话精神,以及《国家中长期教育改革和发展规划纲要(2010—2020)》《中医药发展战略规划纲要(2016—2030年)》和《关于医教协同深化中医药教育改革与发展的指导意见》等文件要求,坚持高等教育立德树人这一根本任务,立足中医药教育改革发展要求,遵循我国中医药事业发展规律和中医药教育规律,深化中医药特色的人文素养和思想情操教育,从而达到以文化人、以文育人的效果。

同时,全国中医药高等教育学会教学管理研究会和上海科学技术出版社将不断深化高等中医药教材研究,在新版精编教材的编写组织中,努力将教材的编写出版工作与中医药发展的现实目标及未来方向紧密联系在一起,促进中医药人才培养与"健康中国"战略紧密结合起来,实现全程育人、全方位育人,不断完善高等中医药教材体系和丰富教材品种,创新、拓展相关课程教材,以更好地适应"十三五"时期及今后高等中医药院校的教学实践要求,从而进一步地提高我国高等中医药人才的培养能力,为建设健康中国贡献力量!

教材的编写出版需要在实践检验中不断完善,诚恳地希望广大中医药院校师生和读者在教学实践或使用中对本套教材提出宝贵意见,以敦促我们不断提高。

全国中医药高等教育学会常务理事、教学管理研究会理事长

胡鸿毅

2016年12月

中医英语课程是中医学、针灸推拿学、中西医临床医学等专业本科生和研究生的一门必修课，其教学宗旨是将英语学习和中医药专业相结合，使学生通过课程学习，掌握中医药基本理论的英语表达与基本翻译技能，提高学生的中医药英语综合应用能力，为学生今后用英语开展中医药临床和科研实践打下坚实的基础。

本教材在充分考虑中医药类专业学生的学习特点和他们未来的职业发展的基础上，努力探索一种基于内容的专业英语教学模式(CBT, Content-based Teaching)，即以中医药专业内容为依托，学习中医药专业的相关英语表达，提高学生专业英语综合应用能力。

本教材在《中医英语》(第2版)的基础上，结合教学实际，共设置10个单元，内容包括中医学概况、中医学核心概念、中医藏象理论、气血精液、病因病机、四诊法则、经络系统、方剂方药、针灸治疗和中医药临床应用。每个单元包括课前热身视听(Warming-up)、主题课文阅读(Text A、Text B)和中医药术语推展，并设计了多样化的练习，具有以下特点。

1. **保留了《中医英语》(第2版)教材的大部分文章**　本教材共选取20篇阅读文章，其中大部分来源于前版教材，其余选编自英美原版资料，这样既保持了教材内容的系统性和连续性，也反映了中医药术语英译和国际标准化的最新进展。

2. **教材结构逻辑设计利于学生学习掌握**　每单元首先是由相关的视听进行引入，随后是单元主题相关的两篇阅读文章，在阅读文章之后是与本单元主题相关的中医药基本术语汇总，练习设计力求从听、说、读、写、译等方面全面培养学生的综合语言技能，注重将学生在中医药领域语言能力和术语能力的训练贯穿始终。每个单元的 Text A 都以脚注形式对文章重点难点进行注释，Text B 的生词都以旁注的形式呈现，方便学生理解课文。

3. **注重培养学生英语应用和批判思维能力**　练习设计形式多样，如在视听热身部分设计了听力填空题型，听力填空后是有关视听主题的主观题，强调学生对于所听内容的主要思想和细节的掌握；随后是单元主题相关的两篇阅读文章，文章练习设计既注重学生对于文章主要意思的理解,又注重对文章细节的掌握,训练和引导学生对于相关主题进行深层次的讨论,帮助学生理解课文内容和掌握相关语言现象。

4. 反映中医药国际交流最新进展　根据世界卫生组织西太区和世界中医药联合会发布的术语标准,每单元设计了与本单元主题相关的中医药术语对比表,在拓展术语翻译的同时,给学生提供术语翻译的不同视角。注重对于中医药相关词汇、句型的总结与考查。每篇课文后面都设计了多项词汇和术语练习,主要是每课出现的与中医药学相关的术语、词汇与句型,题型采取填空、配对、选词填空和翻译等形式,其中选词填空句子大多来源于英美最新的报刊资料。

本书正文后面设有3个附录,附录1为中医典籍英译节选,目的是让同学们了解中医药典籍的翻译;附录2为常用中医药学科和专业人员的英语表达;附录3为世界卫生组织2018年公布的国际疾病分类第11版(ICD‐11)中传统医学章节的中英文术语,反映了中医术语英译及其国际标准化在国内外的最新发展。

5. 融"纸质＋视听＋课件"一体的多模态立体化教材　本教材除了纸质版外,根据课程目标,编制了以扫描二维码作为本课程学习的辅助模式,包括视听内容、课文朗读、参考译文、练习答案、PPT课件等,供师生学习和教学时参考。

本教材是在《中医英语》(第2版)教材的基础上,结合现代专业英语教学理念和中医药翻译学科的进展而进行修订。在此,向前版教材编委会表示诚挚的敬意和感谢,也感谢各兄弟院校对本次教材修订的大力支持。

本教材的编写思路由施建蓉提出,章节体例由周恩制定完成。第一单元和第十单元由施建蓉、周恩、蒋辰雪、苏琳负责编写,第二单元由郭先英、李苹负责编写,第三单元由李晓莉、董俭、王世杰负责编写,第四单元由刘娅、毛和荣、张毓彪负责编写,第五单元由董敏华、扈李娟负责编写,第六单元由范延妮、李成华负责编写,第七单元由徐永红、马白菊负责编写,第八单元由陈骥、赖寒、师旭亮负责编写,第九单元由李涛安、徐立群、罗茜负责编写,最后由施建蓉和周恩对书稿进行统稿、审核和修改。Sean Bradley和丁年青对教材进行了审定。

中医药走向世界,开展对外交流与合作,离不开中医药从业人员的专业外语水平的不断提高。希望本教材能够有助于中医药学生和从业者专业英语水平的提高。由于时间、能力等因素,书中纰缪之处在所难免,敬请广大读者和学界同仁批评指正,以便修订完善。

《中医英语》编委会

2020 年 4 月

本书配套数字教学资源

微信扫描二维码，加入中医英语
读者交流圈，获取配套教学视
频、学习课件、课后习题和沟通交
流平台等板块内容，夯实基础知识

Contents

The great arrangements of heaven and earth,
this is what all men and spirits correspond to.
天地之大纪,人神之通应也①。

Unit 1　Traditional Chinese Medicine: An Introduction

Warming-up

Before you listen (Watch)

In this section you will hear a short passage about "Traditional Chinese Medicine". The following words and phrases may be of help.

Traditional Chinese Medicine (TCM)		中医,中医学
physiology /ˌfɪzɪˈɒlədʒɪ/	*n*.	生理学,生理机能
artemisinin /ˌɑːtɪˈmiːsɪnɪn/	*n*.	青蒿素
malaria /məˈleərɪə/	*n*.	疟疾
stretch back	*v*.	回溯到
inseparable /ɪnˈseprəbl/	*a*.	不可分的
revere /rɪˈvɪə(r)/	*v*.	敬畏,尊敬
acupuncture /ˈækjupʌŋktʃə(r)/	*n*.	针刺
moxibustion /ˌmɒksɪˈbʌstʃ(ə)n/	*n*.	艾灸
massage /ˈmæsɑːʒ/	*n*.	推拿
cupping /ˈkʌpɪŋ/	*n*.	拔罐
therapy /ˈθerəpɪ/	*n*.	治疗,疗法

While you listen(Watch)

Listen to the passage carefully and fill in each of the blanks marked from 1) to 10) according to what you have heard.

In the year 2015, the whole world was rejoicing for a Chinese woman named Tu Youyou

---

① 《素问·至真要大论篇》,Paul U. Unschuld 译。

because using traditional Chinese medicine, she sent a 1) _____ to the world. At the Nobel Prize Award Ceremony where she received the Nobel Prize in Physiology and Medicine, Tu Youyou 2) _____ the world: Traditional Chinese medicine is a vast treasure-house, we really ought to fully explore and improve. She discovered artemisinin, an anti-malaria naturally 3) _____ chemical, through information from this treasure-house. From her research experience with artemisinin, she fully realized when traditional Chinese medicine and modern western medicine are combined in a way that 4) _____ the other, a whole new range of potential and a promising future is opened.

Over the gradual 5) _____ of these thousands of years, traditional Chinese medicine never forgot its principles of adhering to the laws of nature, revering life, balancing *yin* and *yang*, and bringing 6) _____. From this background, traditional Chinese medicine evolved to develop many forms of treatment, such as herbal medicine, acupuncture and moxibustion, Tuina, massage, cupping, Qigong, and food therapy.

Since ancient times, people from all over the world were coming to China and 7) _____ with the culture and knowledge. Now in present times, traditional Chinese medicine has spread to 183 countries and districts with 103 countries already 8) _____ the use of acupuncture, and hundreds of TCM schools spread in over 30 countries. In the year 2015, there were already 3,966 TCM hospitals and 9) _____ clinics in China with the number of 10) _____ visits for the year reaching 910 million.

After you listen(Watch)

Please discuss with your partner the following questions and give your presentation to the class.

1) Why did Tu Youyou win the Noble Prize in Physiology and Medicine?
2) What principles does traditional Chinese medicine adhere to?
3) Please list some forms of treatment in traditional Chinese medicine.
4) What are the differences between traditional Chinese medicine and Western medicine?

Reading

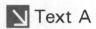 Text A

BEFORE CLASS

1. **Quest for Definition**

Directions: Explore online the definitions of the following terms from Text A and prepare a unique *one-minute* oral presentation for your class.

1) acupuncture and moxibustion
2) syndrome differentiation

3) four properties and five flavors

4) correspondence between man and nature

2. Text-based Activities

Directions: Read carefully the part of Text A that corresponds to your task, and then prepare a unique *one-minute* **oral presentation for your class.**

PERFORMANCE IN CLASS

Your Task

1) How do you define traditional Chinese medicine?

2) What classics of traditional Chinese medicine do you know?

3) Why is the *Huangdi Neijing* considered the greatest classic in traditional Chinese medicine?

4) What are the major contributions to traditional Chinese medicine made respectively by the four great medical schools in the Jin and Yuan Dynasties?

5) Please briefly introduce Li Shizhen and the *Bencao Gangmu* (*Compendium of Materia Medica*) to your class.

Traditional Chinese medicine: History and Development

1   Traditional Chinese medicine (TCM), with a history of thousands of years, unique and integrated theoretical system, rich practical experience and good clinical effect, has been making great contribution to Chinese people's health care and to the development of Chinese nation. It is a summary of the Chinese people's experience in their struggle against diseases. Over the past few decades it has been attracting increasing attention from all over the world.

2   The formation of TCM theoretical system can be traced back to the period of the Warring States and the Qin and Han Dynasties①. During the long course of TCM development, ancient medical experts took ancient Chinese philosophical thinking as the guide, constantly absorbing knowledge from ancient natural and social sciences. The **compilation** of the *Huangdi Neijing* (*Huangdi's Canon of Medicine*), *Nan Jing* (*Classic of Difficulties*), *Shanghan Zabing Lun* (*Treatise on Cold Damage and Miscellaneous Diseases*), and Shennong *Bencao Jing* (*Shennong's Classic of Materia Medica*) ②, known in TCM as the Four Great Classics, is the symbol of the primary formation of the theoretical system of TCM.

---

①   traced back to the period of the Warring States and the Qin and Han Dynasties: (中医学理论体系的形成)可追溯到战国和秦汉时期。

②   *Huangdi Neijing* (*Huangdi's Canon of Medicine*):《黄帝内经》; *Nan Jing* (*Classic of Difficulties*): 《难经》; *Shanghan Zabing Lun* (*Treatise on Cold Damage and Miscellaneous Diseases*):《伤寒杂病论》; *Shennong Bencao Jing* (*Shennong's Classic of Materia Medica*):《神农本草经》。此四书一般被称为中医四大经典。

3　The *Huangdi Neijing*, as the earliest and greatest medical classic **extant** in China, was completed by many medical experts in history. It is so important that even now, after thousands of years, it is still regarded as the most **authoritative** one in TCM. This work consists of two **distinct** books, i. e. the *Su Wen* (*Plain Conversation*) and the *Ling Shu* (*Spiritual Pivot*)①, each comprising nine volumes. The content of the *Huangdi Neijing* covers the following aspects: the correspondence between man and nature②, physiology and pathology of the human body as well as diagnosis, treatment and prevention of diseases. By applying the theories of *yin-yang* and the five elements, it has developed the therapeutic principles based on syndrome differentiation③, seasonal changes, geographical localities and individual **constitution**.

4　The *Nan Jing* was written approximately before the Han Dynasty and, according to the legend, by Qin Yueren, also known as Bian Que. It deals mainly with the basic theory of TCM, including the knowledge of physiology, pathology, **diagnostics** and **therapeutics**. It has **supplemented** what was **unaddressed** in the *Huangdi Neijing* in many respects, especially in pulse **lore** ④.

5　*Shennong Bencao Jing*, the earliest book on materia medica in China, appeared approximately in the Han Dynasty with its authorship unknown. In this classic, 365 kinds of medicine are recorded, among which 252 are herbs, 67 are animal parts and 46 are mineral products. They are divided into three grades according to their properties and effects⑤. Other content concerning **pharmaceutics** analyzed in this classic includes four properties (cold, hot, warm and cool)⑥, five flavors (sour, bitter, sweet, **pungent** and salty)⑦, and seven conditions of **ingredients** in prescriptions (single effect, mutual reinforcement, mutual assistance, mutual restraint, mutual inhibition, mutual antagonism and mutual **suppression**)⑧.

6　The *Shanghan Zabing Lun* was written by Zhang Zhongjing at the end of the Eastern Han Dynasty. In this book, the rich experience on prevention and treatment of diseases before the Eastern Han Dynasty was summed up, and diagnosis and treatment of cold and miscellaneous diseases were dealt with respectively. This book symbolizes the establishment of treatment based on syndrome differentiation in TCM. It was later divided into two parts: the *Shanghan Lun* (*Treatise on Cold Damage*) and the *Jingui Yaolue* (*Synopsis of Golden Chamber*)⑨. Based on the

---

①　the *Su Wen* (*Plain Questions*)《素问》;the *Ling Shu* (*Spiritual Pivot*)《灵枢》。

②　correspondence between man and nature:天人相应。

③　syndrome differentiation:辨证。

④　It has supplemented what was unaddressed in the *Huangdi Neijing* in many respects, especially in pulse lore:它(《难经》)在许多方面,尤其在脉学上,补《黄帝内经》之不足。

⑤　They are divided into three grades according to their properties and effects:根据特性和功效,它们(365 kinds of medicine)被划分为上、中、下三品。

⑥　four properties (cold, hot, warm and cool):(中药)四气(寒、热、温、凉)。

⑦　five flavors (sour, bitter, sweet, pungent and salty):(中药)五味(酸、苦、甘、辛、咸)。

⑧　seven conditions of ingredients in prescriptions (single effect, mutual reinforcement, mutual assistance, mutual restraint, mutual inhibition, mutual antagonism and mutual suppression):(中药)七情(单行、相使、相须、相畏、相杀、相恶、相反)。

⑨　the *Shanghan Lun* (*Treatise on Cold Damage*) and the *Jingui Yaolue* (*Synopsis of Golden Chamber*):《伤寒论》和《金匮要略》。

Four Great Classics, medical experts in different dynasties further enriched and developed the theoretical system of TCM. Huangfu Mi in the Western Jin Dynasty compiled the *Zhenjiu Jiayi Jing* (*A-B Classics of Acupuncture and Moxibustion*)①, which is the earliest extant work dealing exclusively with acupuncture and moxibustion. In 610, Chao Yuanfan compiled the *Zhubing Yuanhou Lun* (*Treatise on Causes and Manifestations of Various Diseases*)②, the earliest **monograph** on **etiology** and symptomatology in China③. In 657, Su Jing, together with 20 other scholars, compiled the *Xinxiu Bencao* (*Newly-Revised Materia Medica*)④, which is the first state-sponsored **pharmacopoeia** in China and the earliest **pharmacopoeia** in the world⑤. Another famous physician Sun Simiao (581 – 682) devoted all his life to the writing of two great books: the *Beiji Qianjin Yaofang* (*Valuable Prescriptions for Emergency*) and the *Qianjin Yifang* (*Supplement to Valuable Prescriptions*)⑥. In the Song Dynasty, more attention was paid to medical education. The government set up "the Imperial Medical Bureau⑦" for training and educating qualified medical workers. In 1057, a special organization named "Bureau for Revising Medical Books⑧" was set up in order to **proofread** and correct the medical books published in previous dynasties.

7　In the Jin and Yuan Dynasties, there appeared four great medical schools represented by⑨ Liu Wansu (1120 – 1200), Zhang Congzheng (1156 – 1228), Li Gao (1180 – 1251) and Zhu Zhenheng (1281 – 1358). Liu Wansu believed that "fire-heat" was the main cause of a variety of diseases and these diseases should be treated with drugs cold and cool in nature. So his theory was known as the "School of Cold and Cool". Zhang Congzheng believed that all diseases were caused by **exogenous pathogenic** factors⑩ and advocated that pathogenic factors should be driven out by means of **diaphoresis**, **emesis** and **purgation**. For this reason, his theory was known as the "School of Purgation". Li Gao held that "internal **impairment** of the spleen and stomach would bring about various diseases" and emphasized that the most important thing in clinical treatment was to warm and **invigorate** the spleen and stomach. Therefore he was regarded as the founder of the "School of Reinforcing the Earth". Zhu Zhenheng believed that "*yang* is usually excessive while *yin* is

---

①　*Zhenjiu Jiayi Jing* (*A-B Classics of Acupuncture and Moxibustion*):《针灸甲乙经》。

②　*Zhubing Yuanhou Lun* (*Treatise on Causes and Manifestations of Various Diseases*):《诸病源候论》。

③　the earliest monograph on etiology and symptomology in China: 它是中国现存最早的病因证候学专著。

④　*Xinxiu Bencao* (*Newly-Revised Materia Medica*):《新修本草》。

⑤　the first state-sponsored pharmacopoeia in China and the earliest pharmacopoeia in the world: 古代中国第一部国家药典和世界最早的药典。

⑥　*Beiji Qianjin Yaofang* (*Valuable Prescriptions for Emergency*) and *Qianjin Yifang* (*Supplement to Valuable Prescriptions*):《备急千金要方》和《千金翼方》。

⑦　the Imperial Medical Bureau: 太医局。

⑧　Bureau for Revising Medical Books: 校正医书局(宋代政府设置,这是我国出版史上首次由政府设立的医书校正专门机构)。

⑨　four great medical schools represented by …: 以……为代表的四大医学流派。即下文的 "the School of Cold and Cool" "寒凉派";"the School of Purgation" "攻下派";"the School of Reinforcing the Earth" "补土派"和"the School of Nourishing *Yin*" "滋阴派"。

⑩　exogenous pathogenic factors: 外邪。

frequently deficient"① and advocated the **remedies** of nourishing *yin* and reducing fire in treatment of disease. That is why his theory was known as the "School of Nourishing *Yin*".

8   Li Shizhen (1518–1593), a famous physician and **pharmacologist** in the Ming Dynasty, wrote *Bencao Gangmu* (*Compendium of Materia Medica*)②. This book consists of 52 volumes in which 1,892 medicinal herbs, over 11,000 prescriptions and 1,100 illustrations of medicinal items are presented. It deals with the knowledge of many subjects, such as **botany**, **zoology**, **mineralogy**, physics, **astronomy** and meteorology. This book is recognized as a **monumental** work in the history of Chinese materia medica③ and a great contribution to the development of pharmacology in the world.

9   Due to severe infectious diseases in the Ming and Qing Dynasties, the school of warm diseases emerged dealing with diagnosis, prevention and treatment of warm diseases.

10   After the Opium War (1840–1842), Western medicine began to **disseminate** in China, exerting certain influence on④ the practice of TCM. Some Chinese medical experts tried to combine TCM with Western medicine. The *Yixue Zhongzhong Canxi Lu* (*Records of Traditional Chinese and Western Medicine in Combination*) written by Zhang Xichun⑤ is a representative monograph in this field.

11   After the founding of the People's Republic of China in 1949, great progress in theoretical study and clinical research of TCM has been made with modern scientific methods and advanced technology by doctors, researchers and other scientists. (1,144 words)

New Words and Expressions

pathogenic /ˌpæθəˈdʒenɪk/ *adj*. something that leads to disease 致病的

miscellaneous /ˌmɪsəˈleɪnɪəs/ *adj*. of mixed sorts; having various qualities and characteristics 各式各样的;杂的

treatise /ˈtriːtɪs/ *n*. a long and serious piece of writing on a particular subject 专著,论文

extant /ekˈstænt/ *adj*. still in existence (esp. of documents, etc.) 现存的

authoritative /ɔːˈθɒrətətɪv/ *adj*. that you can trust and respect as true and correct 权威性的

distinct /dɪsˈtɪŋkt/ *adj*. clearly different or separate 截然不同

pivot /ˈpɪvət/ *n*. central point on which sth. turns 枢轴;支点

constitution /ˌkɒnstɪˈtjuːʃn/ *n*. the condition of a person's body and how healthy it is 身体素质;体质;体格

diagnostics /ˌdaɪəɡˈnɒstɪks/ *n*. the branch of medical science dealing with the identifying the exact cause of disease 诊断学·

---

①   "*Yang* is usually excessive while *yin* is frequently deficient":"阳常有余;阴常不足。"
②   *Bencao Gangmu* (*Compendium of Materia Medica*):《本草纲目》。
③   Chinese materia medica:中药学,也译作 Chinese pharmacy。
④   exerting certain influence on …:对……施加影响。
⑤   *Yixue Zhongzhong Canxi Lu* (*Records of Traditional Chinese and Western Medicine in Combination*) written by Zhang Xichun:张锡纯《医学衷中参西录》。

therapeutics /ˌθerə'pjuːtɪks/ *n*. the branch of medicine concerned with the treatment of disease 治疗学

supplement /'sʌplɪmənt/ *n*. sth. added later to improve or complete (e. g. a dictionary) 附录,增刊; *vt*. to complete, add to, or extend by a supplement 补遗;补充

lore /lɔː/ *n*. the body of knowledge, esp. of a traditional, anecdotal, or popular nature, on a particular subject; learning, knowledge, or erudition 学问,知识

unaddressed /ʌnə'drest/ *adj*. not considered or dealt with 未予考虑的,未解决的

pungent /'pʌndʒənt/ *adj*. having a strong taste or smell 味道(或气味)强烈的;刺激性的

pharmaceutics /ˌfɑːmə'sjuːtɪks/ *n*. the art and science of preparing and dispensing drugs and medicines 制药学

ingredient /ɪn'griːdɪənt/ *n*. one of the things from which sth. is made, especially one of the foods that are used together to make a particular dish 成分;(尤指烹饪)原料

suppression /sə'preʃn/ *n*. forceful prevention; putting down by power or authority 压制;抑制

synopsis /sɪ'nɒpsɪs/ *n*. summary or outline (of a book, play, etc.) 大纲;要略

etiology /ˌiːtɪ'ɒlədʒɪ/ *n*. study of the causes of disease 病源学,病因学

pharmacopoeia /ˌfɑːməkə'piːə/ *n*. (officially published) book with list of medicinal preparations and directions for their use (官方出版的)药典

emergency /ɪ'mɜːdʒənsɪ/ *n*. sudden happening which makes quick action necessary 急诊

gynecology /ˌɡaɪnɪ'kɒlədʒɪ/ *n*. the branch of medicine that deals with the diseases and hygiene of women 妇科学

obstetrics /ɒb'stetrɪks/ *n*. the branch of medicine dealing with childbirth and care of the mother 产科学

pediatrics /ˌpiːdɪ'ætrɪks/ *n*. the branch of medicine concerned with the treatment of infants and children 儿科学

proofread /'pruːfriːd/ *vt*. read and correct proofs 校对;改正校稿

exogenous /ek'sɒdʒɪnəs/ *adj*. of external cause 外因的

diaphoresis /ˌdaɪəfə'riːsɪs/ *n*. perspiration, especially when copious and artificially or medically induced 出汗;发汗

emesis /'eməsɪs/ *n*. vomiting; the reflex act of ejecting the contents of the stomach through the mouth 呕吐;呕吐的行为

purgation /pɜː'ɡeɪʃən/ *n*. purging of the bowels; the use of a cathartic to stimulate evacuation of the bowels 净肠;洗肠;通便

impairment /ɪm'peəmənt/ *n*. the fact that a part of your body is unable to do something fully 缺陷,障碍,损伤

invigorate /ɪn'vɪɡəreɪt/ *v*. to give someone more energy 使生气勃勃;使精神焕发

remedy /'remɪdɪ/ *n*. a medicine or therapy that cures disease or relieve pain 药物,治疗法,补救,赔偿; *vt*. to cure, relieve, or heal 治疗,补救,矫正

pharmacologist /ˌfɑːmə'kɒlədʒɪst/ *n*. expert in pharmacology 药物学家

compendium /kəm'pendɪəm/ *n*. concise and comprehensive account; summary 摘要;概要

botany /'bɒtənɪ/ *n.* the scientific study of plants and their structure 植物学

zoology /zəʊ'ɒlədʒɪ/ *n.* the scientific study of animals and their behavior 动物学

mineralogy /ˌmɪnə'rælədʒɪ/ *n.* the scientific study of minerals 矿物学

astronomy /ə'strɒnəmɪ/ *n.* science of the sun, moon, stars and planets 天文学

anatomy /ə'nætəmɪ/ *n.* the scientific study of the bodies and body parts of people and animal 解剖学

compilation /ˌkɒmpɪ'leɪʃən/ *n.* the act or process of compiling 汇编,编辑

pathogenesis /ˌpæθə'dʒenɪsɪs/ *n.* mechanism involved in the occurrence of disease 发病;发病机制

monumental /ˌmɒnju'mentl/ *adj.* used for emphasizing how good or important something is 重要的;意义深远的

disseminate /dɪ'semɪneɪt/ *v.* spread or disperse (something, especially information) widely 散步,传播,扩散

monograph /'mɒnəɡrɑːf/ *n.* detailed scientific account, esp. a published report on some item of research 专论

FOLLOW-UP ACTIVITIES

Task one   Comprehension Check

1. Questions for Discussion

1) What are the characteristics of traditional Chinese medicine?

2) Please briefly introduce the history and development of traditional Chinese medicine.

3) What contribution has traditional Chinese medicine made to the world medicine?

4) Please search for the information about the global development of TCM.

2. Chart Completion

INTRODUCTION: (para. 1 - 2)

    Traditional Chinese medicine (TCM), with a history of thousands of years, is a summary of the Chinese people's experience in 1) _____ . The 2) _____ can be traced back to the period of 3) _____ .

FOUR CLASSICS: (para. 3 - 6)

    The *Huangdi Neijing*, the earliest and greatest medical classic extant in China, developed the therapeutic principles based on 4) _____ , seasonal changes, geographical localities and individual constitution.

    The *Nan Jing* deals mainly with 5) _____ and has supplemented what was unaddressed in the *Huangdi Neijing* in many respects, especially in 6) _____ .

    The *Shennong Bencao Jing*, the earliest book on materia medica in China, recorded 365 kinds of medicine which are divided into three grades according to 7) _____ , and four properties, five flavors and 8) _____ .

The *Shanghan Zabing Lun* recorded the diagnosis and treatment of 9) _____ ____ . This book symbolizes the establishment of treatment based on syndrome differentiation in TCM.

HISTORY AND DEVELOPMENT: (para. 7 – 11)

The TCM theoretical system was enriched and developed by medical experts, including Huangfu Mi, Chao Yuanfan, Sun Simiao, etc.

In the Song Dynasty, more attention was paid to 10) _____ .

In the Jin and Yuan Dynasties, there appeared 11) _____ represented by Liu Wansu, Zhang Congzheng, Li Gao and Zhu Zhenheng.

In the Ming Dynasty, Li Shizhen (1518 – 1593) wrote the *Bencao Gangmu*, *which* is recognized as a monumental work in the history of 12) _____ .

In the Ming and Qing Dynasties, there emerged the 13) _____ dealing with diagnosis, prevention and treatment of warm diseases.

After the Opium War (1840 – 1842), Western medicine began to disseminate in China. Some Chinese medical experts tried to 14) _____ .

After the founding of the People's Republic of China in 1949, great progress in TCM has been made with 15) _____ by doctors, researchers and other scientists.

Task Two   Vocabulary

1. **Directions: Complete the following phrases respectively according to its corresponding meaning or equivalent in Chinese within the brackets.**

1) _____ (理论的) system

2) ancient Chinese _____ (哲学的) thinking

3) _____ (汇编) of the *Huangdi Neijing*

4) the most _____ (权威的) one

5) the _____ (对应) between man and nature

6) individual _____ (体质)

7) pulse _____ (学问,知识)

8) with its _____ (作者身份) unknown

9) four _____ (属性)

10) seven conditions of _____ (成分)

11) mutual _____ (加强)

12) mutual _____ (帮助)

13) mutual _____ (约束)

14) mutual _____ (抑制)

15) mutual _____ (对立)

16) mutual _____ (废止;压制)

17) _____ (杂的) diseases

18) dealing _____ (仅仅,唯一地) with acupuncture and moxibustion

19) the earliest _____ (现存的) works

20) monograph on _____ (病因学)

21) the first _____ (药典)

22) _____ (药方) for Emergency

23) _____ (校对) medical books

24) _____ (外因的) pathogenic factors

25) internal _____ (损伤)

26) _____ (使精力充沛) the spleen

27) famous _____ (药物学家)

28) _____ (不朽的) work

29) _____ (传染的) diseases

30) representative_____ (专论)

2. Match the following words with their proper meanings.

Column I	Column II
1) authorship	a. a connection between two things
2) integration	b. a drawing or picture in a book, magazine, etc. especially one that explains sth.
3) differentiation	c. to produce a book, list, report, etc. by bringing together different items, articles, songs, etc.
4) impairment	d. The process of combining with other things in a single larger unit or system
5) correspondence	e. very important and having a great influence, especially as the result of years of work
6) disseminate	f. greater than what seems reasonable or appropriate
7) illustration	g. the state of having a physical or mental condition which means that part of your body or brain does not work correctly
8) compile	h. a discrimination between things as different and distinct
9) reinforcement	i. not having enough of sth., especially sth. that is essential
10) invigorate	j. the identity of the person who wrote sth., especially a book
11) monumental	k. the act of restricting or preventing a process or an action
12) deficient	l. forceful prevention
13) inhibition	m. to spread information, knowledge, etc. so that it reaches many people
14) excessive	n. the act of making sth. stronger, especially a feeling or an idea
15) suppression	o. to make sb feel healthy and full of energy

3. Fill in the blanks with the words from the box and change the form when necessary.

integration	illustration	authorship	excessive	impair
compile	disseminate	monumental	invigorate	suppress
reinforce	correspondence	deficient	inhibit	differentiate

1) The study helps us understand how memories are assembled in the brain and how different types of brain damage might _____ memory.

2) The University of Chicago group _____ data on both state and county levels, looking at each area's confirmed cases, deaths and number of cases weighted by population size.

3) "This is a big step forward to _____ and enhance the European social model and cohesion (凝聚力) for the future," he said.

4) First _____ is important to consider because first authors perform a significantly higher proportion of research publication-related tasks than all other authors.

5) Cancer campaigners are hailing (称赞;欢迎) a "_____ leap forward" in pancreatic (胰腺的) cancer treatment after a new drug trial significantly extended survival from what is the most lethal form of the disease.

6) They suggest that technologies like artificial intelligence and self-driving cars will soon accelerate productivity growth and _____ the economy.

7) It is usually difficult for a doctor to _____ between a malignant and benign polyp (恶性和良性的息肉) by appearance, so they will usually remove it during the exam.

8) The Belt and Road Initiative is a Beijing-led program aimed at boosting economic _____ through infrastructure and energy investments in Asia and beyond.

9) There is a definite _____ between infant mortality and poverty.

10) _____ sunlight can lead to freckles (雀斑) or other skin changes, some of which can be detrimental (有害的).

11) It's possible that one lockdown might not be enough, and severe efforts to _____ the virus might be needed again, he says.

12) Over the past few years, investigators have discovered small molecules (分子) that normally stimulate or _____ these responses in the body.

13) He emphasized ways to visualize knowledge and he pioneered anatomical _____.

14) The researchers found virus genetic material on commonly used items such as toilets, but also in air samples, thus indicating that "SARS - CoV - 2 is widely _____ in the environment."

15) Yet one-third of food is wasted, 800 million people remain undernourished, 2 billion are _____ in micronutrients (微量营养元素), and obesity is on the rise.

Task Three   Translation

1   Translate the following medical expressions into English

1) 中国医药学

2) 中医基础理论

3) 临床经验

4) 辨证论治

5) 杂病

6) 中药学

7) 四气五味

8) 针灸

9) 古代中国哲学

10) 汗法

11) 下法

12) 吐法

13) 补土派

14) 病因学

15) 方剂
16) 医疗实践
17) 治疗原则
18) 寒凉药物
19) 滋阴降火
20) 瘀血致病

2　Translate the following sentences into Chinese or English

1) Traditional Chinese medicine (TCM), with a history of thousands of years, is a summary of the Chinese people's experience in their struggle against diseases.

2) Liu Wansu believed that "fire-heat" was the main cause of a variety of diseases and these diseases should be treated with drugs cold and cool in nature.

3) Zhang Congzheng believed that all diseases were caused by exogenous pathogenic factors and advocated that pathogenic factors should be driven out by means of diaphoresis, emesis and purgation.

4) Li Gao, entitled with the School of Reinforcing the Earth, emphasized on warming and invigorating the spleen and stomach.

5) Internal impairment of the spleen and stomach would bring about various diseases.

6) 世界卫生组织将以中医药为主体的传统医学纳入新版国际疾病分类(ICD‐11)。(include)

7) 中国政府致力于推动国际传统医药发展。(devote to)

8) 中医药不仅为中华民族繁衍昌盛做出了卓越贡献,也对世界文明进步产生了积极影响。(exert … influence on)

9) 专利最早可以追溯到 15 世纪的威尼斯。(be traced back to)

10) 温病学派创立了以卫气营血和三焦为核心的温病辨证论治规范。(develop … based on)

3　Translate the following passage into English

　　中医药在历史发展进程中,兼容并蓄、创新开放,形成了独特的生命观、健康观、疾病观、防治观,实现了自然科学与人文科学的融合和统一,蕴含了中华民族深邃的哲学思想。随着人们健康观念变化和医学模式转变,中医药越来越显示出独特价值。

↘ Text B

The Basic Characteristics of TCM Theoretical System

1　The theoretical system of traditional Chinese medicine (TCM) has evolved in the long course of clinical practice under the guidance of classical Chinese **materialism** and **dialectics**. It originates from practice and, in turn, guides the practice. This unique theoretical system is essentially **characterized** by the concept of holism and treatment based on syndrome differentiation.

Concept of holism

2　The concept of **holism** is a reflection of classical Chinese

materialism /məˈtɪərɪəlɪzəm/ n. 唯物主义

dialectics /ˌdaɪəˈlektɪks/ n. 辩证法

characterize /ˈkærɪktəraɪz/ v. 具有……特点

holism /ˈhəʊlɪzm/ n. 整体论

materialism and dialectics in TCM, emphasizing the **integrity** of the human body and the unity between the body and its external environments. The holism **permeates** through the physiology, pathology, diagnostics, syndrome differentiation and therapeutics.

3   The human body is regarded as an organic whole. Its **constituent** parts are inseparable in structure, **interdependent** in physiology, and mutually influential in pathology. The unity of the body is realized through the five *zang*-organs, with the assistance of the six *fu*-organs and the communication of the **meridian** system. Since the human body is an organic whole, treatment of a local disease in TCM has to take the whole body into consideration. For example, the heart opens into the tongue and is related to the small intestine internally and externally. Given this correlation, oral **erosion** (**ulcerative stomatitis**) may be clinically treated by clearing away the fire from the heart or small intestine. There are a number of therapeutic principles in TCM developed under the guidance of the concept of organic whole, such as "drawing *yin* from *yang* and drawing *yang* from *yin*; treating the right for curing disease located in the left, treating the left for curing disease located in the right"; "needling the acupoints on the lower part of the body for the treatment of the disease located in the upper part, and needling the acupoints on the upper part of the body for the treatment of the disease located in the lower part."

4   Man lives in the natural world and the natural world provides man with all the necessities **indispensable** to his existence. At the same time, the changes in nature directly or indirectly affect the human body. Take seasonal changes as an example, usually spring is marked by warmth, summer by heat, late summer by dampness, autumn by dryness and winter by cold. Under the influence of such changes, the living things on the earth change to adapt to environmental variation, such as **sprouting** in spring, growing in summer, transforming in late summer, ripening in autumn and storage in winter. The human body is no exception and also makes corresponding changes to adapt to the changing seasons. For example, in spring and summer, *yang qi* goes outward and flourishes, and *qi* and blood of the body tend to circulate superficially, consequently leading to more sweating and less urination. While during autumn and winter, *yang qi* goes inward and **astringes**, *qi* and blood of the body tend to flow internally,

integrity /ɪnˈtegrɪtɪ/ *n*. 完整

permeate /ˈpɜːmɪeɪt/ *v*. 渗透；弥漫；扩散

constituent /kənˈstɪtjʊənt/ *adj*. 组成的，构成的；*n*. 成分，要素

interdependent /ˌɪntədɪˈpendənt/ *adj*. 相互依存的，相互依赖的

meridian /məˈrɪdɪən/ *n*. 子午线；经线（在中医上指"经脉"）

erosion /ɪˈrəʊʒən/ *n*. 腐蚀，糜烂

ulcerative /ˈʌlsərətɪv/ *adj*. 溃疡的；形成溃疡的

stomatitis /ˌstəʊməˈtaɪtɪs/ *n*. 口腔炎

indispensable /ˌɪndɪˈspensəbl/ *adj*. 不可或缺的；必不可少的

sprout /spraʊt/ *v*. 发芽；抽芽；抽条；生长

astringe /əsˈtrɪndʒ/ *vt*. 使收缩，使收敛

causing less sweating and more urination. In this way, the body keeps its balance of water **metabolism** and avoids over consumption of *yang qi*.

metabolism /mə'tæbəlɪzəm/ *n.* 新陈代谢

Treatment based on syndrome differentiation

5　Treatment based on syndrome differentiation, another important feature of the theoretical system of TCM, is a basic principle in TCM for understanding and treating diseases. Syndrome is the **generalization** of the progress of a disease at a certain stage. Since it involves the location, cause and nature of the disease, and the relation between pathogenic factors and healthy *qi*, syndrome can comprehensively and accurately reveal the nature of the disease. Syndrome differentiation implies that the clinical data of a patient collected through the four examinations are analyzed and generalized to **identify** the pathological mechanism of the disease. Treatment means to select the corresponding therapy according to the result of syndrome differentiation. Taken as a whole, treatment based on syndrome differentiation is a process to understand and resolve a disease.

generalization /ˌdʒenrəlaɪ'zeɪʃn/ *n.* 概括；归纳

identify /aɪ'dentɪfaɪ/ *v.* 确认，证明（某事物）；鉴别出（系某人或某物）

6　TCM emphasizes syndrome differentiation, because only when the syndrome is accurately differentiated can a correct treatment be provided. Take common cold for example, its symptoms of fever, **aversion** to cold and pain in the head and body indicate that the disease is in the exterior. However, it is usually differentiated into two syndromes: common cold due to wind-cold and common cold due to wind-heat. For the treatment of the former syndrome in common cold, herbs pungent in taste and warm in nature are used; while for the treatment of the latter syndrome, herbs pungent in taste and cool in nature are used. So accurate differentiation of syndrome is the **prerequisite** for determination of a proper treatment. The core of treatment based on syndrome differentiation is to understand the relation between the nature and manifestation of a disease.

aversion /ə'vɜːʃn/ *n.* 厌恶，憎恶

prerequisite /ˌpriː'rekwəzɪt/ *n.* 先决条件，前提

7　Two important ideas arise from the concept that syndrome is the summary of pathological changes of a disease at a certain stage of its course. The first idea is "treating the same disease with different therapies", which means that one disease may manifest different syndromes at different stages or under different conditions, and thus needs to be treated by different therapies.

Take **measles** for example, the treatment for it varies from stage to stage. The treatment focuses on promoting **eruption** at the early stage because it is not fully erupted, clearing away heat from the lung at the middle stage because lung heat is **exuberant**, and nourishing *yin* to clear away heat at the advanced stage because the heat still **lingers** and the lung and stomach *yin* is consumed. The other idea is "treating different diseases with the same therapy", which means that different diseases may present the same syndrome because they are of the same pathological mechanism, and thus may be treated with the same therapy. For example, **proctoptosis** due to prolonged **dysentery** and **hysteroptosis** are two different diseases. But if they **manifest** the same syndrome of middle *qi* **collapse**, both of them can be treated by lifting middle *qi*.

8　Thus, it can be seen that the treatment of disease in TCM does not simply concentrate on the difference or similarity of diseases, but on the difference or similarity of pathogenesis. This indicates that diseases with the same pathogenesis can be treated with the same therapeutic methods, while diseases with different pathogenesis have to be treated with different therapeutic methods. Such a therapeutic principle is the gist of treatment based on syndrome differentiation. (1,049 words)

measles /ˈmiːzlz/ *n*. 麻疹
eruption /ɪˈrʌpʃən/ *n*. (斑疹等)突然在皮肤上出现；出疹
exuberant /ɪgˈzjuːbərənt/ *adj*. (指植物等)茁壮的，茂盛的，繁茂的
linger /ˈlɪŋgə/ *v*. 逗留；徘徊；拖沓

proctoptosis /ˌprɒktɒpˈtəʊsɪs/ *n*. 直肠脱垂；脱肛
dysentery /ˈdɪsəntrɪ/ *n*. 痢疾
hysteroptosis /ˌhɪstərɒpˈtəʊsɪs/ *n*. 子宫脱垂
manifest /ˈmænɪfest/ *v*. 表明，清楚显示
collapse /kəˈlæps/ *n*. 垮；崩溃；衰落

Notes：

1. The theoretical system of TCM has evolved in the long course of clinical practice under the guidance of classical Chinese materialism and dialectics. 中医学的理论体系是经过长期的临床实践，在唯物论和辩证法思想指导下逐步形成的。

2. It has originated from practice and, in turn, guides the practice. 它(中医学的理论体系)来源于实践，反过来指导实践。

3. concept of holism：整体观。

4. treatment based on syndrome differentiation 辨证论治。

5. The concept of holism is a reflection of classical Chinese materialism and dialectics in TCM, emphasizing the integrity of the human body and the unity between the body and the internal environments. 这一独特理论体系是中国古代唯物论和辩证法在中医学上的反映，它强调人体的整体性及其与外部环境的统一性。

6. The unity of the body is realized through the five *zang*-organs, with the assistance of the six *fu*-organs and the communication of the meridian system. 机体整体统一性是以五脏为中心，配以六腑，经络系统的联系作用而实现的。

7. take ... into consideration 顾及，考虑到……

8. The heart opens into the tongue and is internal-externally related to the small intestine. Given this correlation oral erosion (ulcerative stomatitis) may be clinically treated by clearing away the fire from the heart or small intestine. 心开窍于舌,心与小肠相表里,所以可用清心火或泻小肠火的方法治疗口舌糜烂。

9. "drawing *yin* from *yang* and drawing *yang* from *yin*; treating the right for curing disease in the left, treating the left for curing disease in the right"; "needling the acupoints on the lower part of the body for the treatment of the disease located in the upper part, and needling the acupoints on the upper part of the body for the treatment of the disease located in the lower part". "从阳引阴,从阴引阳;以右治左,以左治右";"病在上者下取之,病在下者高取之"。

10. Man lives in the natural world and the natural world provides man with all the necessities to his existence. 人类生活在自然界中,自然界提供给人类赖以生存的必要条件。

11. spring is marked by warmth, summer by heat, late summer by dampness, autumn by dryness and winter by cold 春温、夏热、长夏湿、秋燥、冬寒。

12. Under the influence of such changes, the living things on the earth will also change to adapt to environmental variation, such as sprouting in spring, growing in summer, transforming in late summer, ripening in autumn and storage in winter. 生物在这种(气候)变化的影响下,就会有春生、夏长、长夏化、秋收、冬藏等适应性的变化。

13. in spring and summer, *yang qi* goes outward and flourishes, and *qi* and blood of the body tend to circulate superficially 春夏阳气升发在外,气血易浮于体表。

14. during autumn and winter, *yang qi* goes inward and astringes, and *qi* and blood of the body tend to flow internally 秋冬阳气收敛内藏,气血闭于内。

15. In this way the body keeps its balance of water metabolism and avoids over consumption of *yang qi*. 这样,机体保持自身的水液代谢平衡,并避免阳气过度消耗。

16. Syndrome is the generalization of a disease at a certain stage in its course of development.证是机体在疾病发展过程中的某一阶段的病理概括。

17. Since it involves the location, cause and nature of the disease, and the relation between pathogenic factors and healthy *qi*, syndrome can comprehensively and accurately reveal the nature of the disease. 由于证包括了病变的部位、原因、性质,以及邪正关系,因而它能更全面、更正确地揭示疾病的本质。

18. TCM emphasizes syndrome differentiation, because only when the syndrome is accurately differentiated can a correct treatment be provided. 中医强调辨证,因为只有准确辨证,才能有合适的疗法。

19. aversion to cold 恶寒

20. Common cold due to wind-cold and common cold due to wind-heat. 风寒感冒和风热感冒。

21. herbs pungent in taste and warm in nature 辛温中(草)药

22. herbs pungent in taste and cool in nature 辛凉中(草)药

23. treating the same disease with different therapies 同病异治

24. treating different diseases with the same therapy 异病同治

25. clearing away heat from the lung 清肺热

26. middle *qi* collapse 中气下陷
27. Such a therapeutic principle is the gist of treatment based on syndrome differentiation. 这一治疗原则就是辨证论治的精神实质。

Task One   Reading Comprehension

1. Which of the following is one of the characteristics of TCM?
   A. Materialism.   B. Dialectics.
   C. Concept of holism.   D. Therapeutics.

2. According to TCM theory, what is／are the most important in the organic whole of the body?
   A. The five *zang*-organs.   B. The meridian system.
   C. The heart.   D. The kidney.

3. According to the concept of holism in TCM, all sayings are correct about the changes of human body EXCEPT _____ .
   A. *yang qi* flourishes in spring and summer
   B. *qi*-blood of the body tends to go and circulate superficially in spring and summer
   C. *yang qi* goes outward during autumn and winter
   D. *qi*-blood of the body tends to go internally during autumn and winter

4. Which one of the following do you think a TCM doctor generally pays more attention to?
   A. Disease.   B. Syndrome.   C. Symptom.   D. Sign.

5. Why different diseases can be treated with the same therapy?
   A. Because different diseases may have different syndromes.
   B. Because different diseases may have the same syndrome.
   C. Because different diseases may have the same cause.
   D. Because different diseases may have the same symptoms.

Task Two   Vocabulary

1. **Directions: Complete the following phrases respectively according to its corresponding meaning or equivalent in Chinese within the brackets.**

   1) classical Chinese _____ (唯物主义)
   2) classical Chinese _____ (辩证法)
   3) concept of _____ (整体观)
   4) _____ (完整) of the human body
   5) the heart _____ (开窍于) the tongue
   6) _____ (不可缺少的) to his existence
   7) circulate _____ (表面地)
   8) water _____ (新陈代谢)
   9) _____ (致病的) factors
   10) _____ (病理学的) mechanism

11) _____ (厌恶) to cold

12) _____ (辛辣的) in taste

13) the _____ (先决条件) for determination

14) _____ (表现) of a disease

15) take _____ (麻疹) for example

16) promoting _____ (出疹) at the early stage

17) _____ (茂盛的) lung heat

18) prolonged _____ (痢疾)

19) middle *qi* _____ (下陷)

20) _____ (要旨) of treatment

2. Fill in the blanks with the words from the box and change the form when necessary.

prerequisite	inseparable	characterize	eruption	integrity
astringe	dysentery	geographical	exuberant	aversion
essential	ulcerative	constituent	interdependent	manifest

1) I think it's especially important for those of us who believe in — in a world where we're _____, mutual interest and mutual respect between nations.

2) They recommend that formal training in research _____ should start at the undergraduate level.

3) The World Health Organization says it wanted a name that did not refer to a _____ location, an animal, an individual or group of people but was "pronounceable and related to the disease."

4) There is no clear evidence that diet has any effect on the treatment of _____ colitis (结肠炎).

5) Thus, while individual investors are comparatively more optimistic, it would be a mistake to describe them as _____.

6) His illness began to _____ itself around this time.

7) The outbreak of an epidemic is something like a natural disaster — a spontaneous, accidental _____ that is no one's fault.

8) We know that in an economy as competitive as ours, an education is a _____ for success.

9) The 2006 Human Development Report, released Thursday in South Africa, says most of the deaths are caused by diarrhea and _____ brought on by dirty water.

10) At its worst it becomes something even more concerning: biophobia (生物恐惧症), the fear of living things and a complete _____ to nature.

11) In an age of nuclear weapons, cyberattacks, terrorism and environmental crises, national security is becoming _____ from global security.

12) The main _____ of wine are acid, tannin (丹宁酸), alcohol, and sugar.

13) The products of our factory are chiefly _____ by their fine workmanship and durability.

14) Stay home unless you must travel for _____ needs such as groceries, pharmaceuticals, medical care, work and limited exercise.

15) It can effectively improve skin quality, whiten skin, improve skin color, _____ pores (毛孔), and leave skin tender, fair and elastic (有弹性的).

Task Three   Writing

Please rewrite the text in a form of abstract (about 150 words)

Terminology

Basic Terminology of TCM Theory

Terminology	WHO[i]	WFCMS[ii]
中医学	traditional Chinese medicine	Chinese medicine; traditional Chinese medicine (TCM)
中药	Chinese medicinal	Chinese materia medica; Chinese medicinal
中医诊断学	traditional Chinese diagnostics	diagnostics of Chinese medicine
中西医结合	integration of traditional Chinese and Western medicine	integration of Chinese and Western medicine
阴阳学说	*yin-yang* theory	*yin-yang* theory
阴阳对立	opposition of *yin* and *yang*	opposition of *yin* and *yang*
五行	five phases	five elements; five phases
整体观念	holism	concept of holism
五脏	five viscera	five *zang*-organs
六腑	six bowels	six *fu*-organs
辛温	pungent-warm	pungent-warm
辛凉	pungent-cool	pungent-cool
七情	seven emotions	seven emotions; seven relations of medicinal compatibility
相须	mutual reinforcement	mutual reinforcement
相使	mutual assistance	mutual assistance
相畏	mutual restraint	mutual restraint
相恶	mutual inhibition	mutual inhibition
相反	antagonism	antagonism
相杀	mutual suppression	mutual suppression
方剂学	formula study	Chinese medical formulas
内经	Internal Classic	Internal Classic
素问	*Plain Questions*	*Plain Questions*
灵枢	*Miraculous Pivot*	*Miraculous Pivot*; *Spiritual Pivot*
伤寒论	*Treatise on Cold Damage Diseases*	*Treatise on Cold Damage Diseases*; *Treatise on Cold Damage*

continued

Terminology	WHO[i]	WFCMS[ii]
温病	warm diseases	warm diseases
本草	materia medica	materia medica
火	fire	fire
火热证	fire-heat pattern/syndrome	fire-heat syndrome/pattern
药性	nature of medicinals	medicinal property
温补脾胃	warm and tonify the spleen and stomach	warming and tonifying spleen and stomach
开窍	open the orifices	resuscitation; opening orifice
清心火	clear heart fire	clearing heart fire
清肺火	clear lung fire	clearing lung fire
口疮	aphtha	aphtha
正气	healthy *qi*	healthy *qi*
邪气	pathogen	pathogenic *qi*
病机	mechanism of disease	mechanism of disease; pathogenesis
发热	fever	fever
虚	deficiency	deficiency
实	excess	excess
表	exterior	exterior
里	interior	interior
表里俱热	heat in both exterior and interior	dual exterior and interior heat
表邪入里	exterior pathogen entering the interior	inward penetration of exterior pathogen
扶正解表	reinforce the healthy *qi* and release the exterior	reinforcing healthy *qi* and relieving exterior
风寒	wind-cold	wind-cold
风热	wind-heat	wind-heat
寒凝气滞	*qi* stagnation due to cold congealing	congealing cold and *qi* stagnation
中气下陷	sunken middle *qi*	sinking of middle *qi*
升举中气	upraise the middle *qi*	raising middle *qi*

注：i. 指世界卫生组织（World Health Organization）西太区 2007 年发布的《WHO 西太平洋地区传统医学名词术语国际标准》（*WHO International Standard Terminologies on Traditional Medicine in the Western Pacific Region*）
ii. 指世界中医药学会联合会（World Federation of Chinese Medicine Societies）2007 年发布的《中医基本名词术语中英对照国际标准》（*International Standard Chinese-English Basic Nomenclature of Chinese Medicine*）

本书配套数字教学资源

微信扫描二维码，加入中医英语
读者交流圈，获取配套教学视
频、学习课件、课后习题和沟通交
流平台等板块内容，夯实基础知识

Yin and *Yang* serve as the Dao（law）of the heavens and the earth，the fundamental principle of all things，the parents of change，the beginning of birth and death and the storehouse of Shenming.

阴阳者,天地之道也,万物之纲纪,变化之父母,
生杀之本始,神明之府也①。

Unit 2　Philosophical Concepts of Traditional Chinese Medicine

Warming-up

Before you listen（Watch）

In this section you will hear a short passage about "*Yin* and *Yang*". The following words and phrases may be of help.

literally /ˈlɪtərəlɪ/	*adv*.	照字面地;逐字地
philosophy /fəˈlɒsəfɪ/	*n*.	哲学
interchangeable /ˌɪntəˈtʃeɪndʒəbl/	*a*.	可互换的
deficiency /dɪˈfɪʃnsɪ/	*n*.	不足;(在中医上)虚
excess /ɪkˈses/	*n*	过量;(在中医上)实
proportioned /prəˈpɔːʃənd/	*a*.	相称的;成比例的

While you listen（Watch）

Listen to the passage carefully and fill in each of the blanks marked from 1）to 10）according to what you have heard.

Hello! We can continue our discussion on traditional Chinese medicine concepts by discussing *yin* and *yang* theory. *Yin* and *yang* literally mean shadow and light. It's a concept that everything in nature is whole and a 1）_____ of *yin* and *yang* energy. It first appeared in the 6th century BC in the *Book of Changes* known as the *I-Ching*. It's a 2）_____ philosophy and it's not

① 《素问·阴阳应象大论篇》,李照国译。

religious, but based on the observations of nature. *Yin* and *yang* theory is the 3) _____ foundation of the entire universe.

Everything in nature is a balance of 4) _____ forces. And these forces are neither good nor bad, but they're just necessary to the existence of everything. *Yang* energy is considered to be male, hot, dry, bright, active, hard, moving, and it's associated with sun and the daytime and summertime. *Yin* energy is considered to be female, cool, wet, dark, quiet, soft, still and it's associated with the moon, night time and winter.

There are three major concepts in *yin* and *yang* theory. The first is opposition. *Yin* and *yang* are opposite 5) _____ to each other. So for example, ice is cold relative to boiling water. The second concept is that they are 6) _____, so one cannot exist without the other. For example, you can't have activity without rest. You will always have *yin* within *yang* and *yang* within *yin*. That's what the two dots in a *yin-yang* symbol represent. The third concept is the idea of transforming and 7) _____. So *yin* turns into *yang*, and *yang* turns into *yin*. And this cycle repeats itself over and over. For example, summer turns into winter and winter turns into summer. There are six major imbalances of *yin* and *yang*. They are *yang* 8) _____ and *yin* deficiency, *yin* and *yang* deficiency, *yang* excess, *yin* excess, and *yin* and *yang* excess. And these all show up differently in the body.

The word "balance" is used a lot in Chinese medicine, but balance is different from harmony. Balance is the first step toward harmony and harmony is an ever-changing state of balance. When two elements are in harmony, their energies are not just equally 9) _____, but they are blended together into a seamless whole. This is a very interesting concept and we will probably discuss this more in the future. To be in harmony, you must balance the *yin* and *yang* energy in the body and in your 10) _____. So you can look at your health and ask yourself: do you have more *yang* energy or more *yin* energy? And then look at your lifestyle: is it more *yin* in nature or *yang* in nature? Understanding this can help you find more balance and then consequently harmony in life. Thanks so much for watching.

After you listen(Watch)

Please discuss with your partner the following questions and give your presentation to the class.

1) What is the original meaning of *yin* and *yang*?
2) What are four major contents in *yin*-*yang* theory?
3) Can you describe the "*Yin*-*yang* Figure" (Taijitu)?
4) Do you have more *yang* energy or more *yin* energy? How do you know it?

Reading

 Text A

BEFORE CLASS

1. Quest for Definition

Directions: Explore online the definitions of the following terms from Text A and prepare a unique *one-minute* **oral presentation for your class.**

1) the opposition between *yin* and *yang*

2) the waning and waxing between *yin* and *yang*

3) the characteristics of five elements

4) the subjugation of five elements

5) the counter-restriction of five elements

2. Text-based Activities

Directions: Read carefully the part of Text A that corresponds to your task, and then prepare a unique *one-minute* **oral presentation for your class.**

PERFORMANCE IN CLASS

Your Task

1) Please list some examples of *yin* and *yang*.
2) How is *yin-yang* theory used to generalize the properties, flavors and actions of medicinal herbs?
3) What are the laws of movements of five elements?
4) Please tell the order of generation of the five elements.
5) Please tell the order of restriction of the five elements.

Philosophical Concepts of Traditional Chinese Medicine

1　The **philosophical** concepts of traditional Chinese medicine reflect a primitive concept of materialism and dialectics and have played an active role in promoting the development of natural sciences in China. In the ancient times, these philosophical concepts were applied to the field of medicine and greatly influenced the establishment and development of TCM.

Concept of *Yin* and *Yang* of TCM

2　*Yin* and *yang* are the summary of the attributes of two opposite aspects of interrelated things or phenomena in nature①. The early connotations of *yin* and *yang* were quite simple, the side facing the sun being *yang* and the reverse side being *yin*②. In the course of their everyday life and work, ancient Chinese people came to understand that all aspects of the natural world could be seen as having a **dual** aspect, for example, day and night, brightness and dimness, movement and stillness, upward and downward directions, heat and cold, etc. Thus, the terms of *yin* and *yang* are used to express these dual and opposite qualities. The best example for the two primary opposite aspects of a contradiction is the relation between water and fire as described in the *Su Wen* that "water and fire are the symbols of *yin* and *yang*."③

3　*Yin* and *yang* oppose each other. The opposition between *yin* and *yang* means that all things or phenomena in the natural world have two opposite aspects known as *yin* and *yang*, such as heaven and earth, motion and quiescence, ascending and descending, **exiting** and entering, etc. The former belongs to *yang* and the latter to *yin* in each pair mentioned above. The unity is the result of mutual opposition and restriction between *yin* and *yang*. Without opposition, there would be no unity; without mutual opposition, there would be no mutual **complementation**. It is just through this kind of opposition and restriction that a dynamic **equilibrium** can be established.

4　*Yin* and *yang* depend on each other. *Yin* and *yang* are opposed to and, at the same time, depend on each other. Neither can exist in **isolation**. In other words, without *yin* there would be no *yang*, and vice versa. When the interdependent relationships between substances, between functions as well as between substances and functions get abnormal, life activities will be broken, thus bringing about **dissociation** of *yin* and *yang*, **depletion** of **essence**, and even an end of life.

5　*Yin* and *yang* **wane** and **wax** between each other. *Yin* and *yang* coexist in a dynamic equilibrium in which one waxes while the other wanes. In other words, waning of *yin* will lead to waxing of *yang* and vice versa. If this relationship goes beyond normal limits, the relative balance of *yin* and *yang* will not be maintained, consequently resulting in either excess or deficiency of *yin* or *yang* and subsequently the occurrence of disease.

6　*Yin* and *yang* transform into each other. Under given conditions, either *yin* or *yang* may transform into its counterpart. That is to say *yin* may be transformed into *yang* and *yang* into *yin*. So it is said in the *Su Wen* that "extreme *yin* turns into *yang*, and extreme *yang* turns into *yin*" and "extreme cold brings on heat, and extreme heat brings on cold". Pathologically, *yin* syndromes can be transformed into *yang* ones, and vice versa.

Concept of Five Elements of TCM

7　The five elements refer to wood, fire, earth, metal and water as well as their motion and changes in the natural world. In the long course of living and working, the ancient Chinese people

①　*Yin* and *yang* are the summary of the attributes of two opposite aspects of interrelated things or phenomena in nature：阴阳是对自然界相互关联的某些事物和现象对立双方的概括。
②　the side facing the sun being *yang* and the reverse side being *yin*：向日为阳,背日为阴。
③　Water and fire are the symbols of *yin* and *yang*：水火者,阴阳之征兆也。

came to understand that these five categories of substances are the most essential and indispensable to their existence.

8   The concept of the five elements holds that all phenomena in the universe correspond in nature either to wood, fire, earth, metal or water, and that these elements are in a state of constant motion and change. In traditional Chinese medicine, the concept of five elements is used to generalize and explain the nature of the *zang-fu* organs, the interrelations among these organs as well as the relationship between human beings and the natural world.

9   According to this concept, everything in nature is attributed to one of the five elements. For instance, wood is characterized by growing freely and **peripherally** ①. So anything with the functions of growing and developing freely is attributed to the category of wood. Fire is characterized by flaming up②. Thereby anything with the functions of warming and rising is attributed to the category of fire. Earth is characterized by cultivation and reaping③. So anything with the functions of generating, transforming, supporting and receiving is attributed to the category of earth. Metal is characterized by change④. Hence anything with the functions of purifying, descending and astringing is attributed to the category of metal. Water is characterized by moistening and downward flowing⑤. Therefore, anything with the functions of cooling, moistening and moving downward is attributed to the category of water.

10   The movement of the five elements is mainly characterized by generation, restriction, **subjugation**, counter-restriction, and mutual interaction between each other.

11   Generation means that one kind of object generates, strengthens or brings forth another⑥, i. e., wood generates fire, fire generates earth, earth generates metal, metal generates water, and water, in turn, generates wood. Each of the five elements is marked by such relations as "being generated" and "generating"⑦. This relationship of the five elements is termed as the "mother-child" relationship. Each element is the "child" of the element that generates it and the "mother" of the one it generates⑧. Take wood for example. Since wood generates fire, it is the mother of fire; because wood is also generated by water, so it is the "child" of water.

12   Restriction implies bringing under control or restraint. The restricting activity among the five elements follows a circular order: wood restricts earth, earth restricts water, water restricts fire, fire restricts metal, and metal, in turn, restricts wood. In this circular order, each of the five

---

①   wood is characterized by growing freely and peripherally：木曰曲直。
②   Fire is characterized by flaming up：火曰炎上。
③   Earth is characterized by cultivation and reaping：土爱稼穑。
④   Metal is characterized by change：金曰从革。
⑤   Water is characterized by moistening and downward flowing：水曰润下。
⑥   Generation means that one kind of object generates, strengthens or brings forth another：相生指这一事物对另一事物具有促进、助长和资生的作用。
⑦   Each of the five elements is marked by such relations as "being generated" and "generating"：对于五行中的任何一"行"来说，都存在着"生我"和"我生"的关系。
⑧   Each element is the "child" of the element that generates it and the "mother" of the one it generates：每一行既是"我生"之"子"，又是"生我"之"母"。

elements is marked by "being restricted" and "restricting"①. For example, the element restricting wood is metal, and the element that is restricted by wood is earth.

13   Subjugation is similar to launching an attack when a counterpart is weak. It is excessive restriction among the five elements. For instance, wood normally restricts earth. However, if wood is in excess, it may over-restrict earth and brings on insufficiency of earth. This is known as wood subjugating earth②. The order of subjugation is the same as that of restriction. Subjugation is not a normal restriction but a harmful condition occurring under abnormal circumstances.

14   Counter-restriction refers to the idea of the strong one bullying the weak③. Among the five elements it implies that one element preys another. It is a morbid condition in which one element fails to restrict the other in the regular order, but is restricted by the other in the reverse order. So the direction of counter-restriction is just the opposite to that of restriction. For example, under normal conditions, metal restricts wood. But when wood is in excess or metal is in deficiency, wood will counter-restrict metal instead of being restricted by metal, which is known as "wood counter-restricting metal④".

15   On the whole, the philosophical concepts of *yin-yang* and five elements permeate through all aspects of the theoretical system of TCM. When applied into TCM, they serve to explain the organic structure, physiological function and pathological changes of the human body, and in addition, guide clinical diagnosis and treatment. (1,231 words)

New Words and Expressions

philosophical /ˌfɪləˈsɒfɪkl/ *adj*. connected with philosophy 哲学的

dual /ˈdjuːəl/ *adj*. having two parts or aspects; double 两部分的；双的；双重的

exit /ˈeksɪt, -zɪt/ *v*. go out; leave 离去；退去

complementation /ˌkɒmplɪmenˈteɪʃn/ *n*. something that goes well or suitably with sth. else, or makes it complete 相匹配的事物；补充物；补足物

equilibrium /ˌiːkwɪˈlɪbrɪəm/, /ˌekwɪˈlɪbrɪəm/ *n*. a state of balance 平衡状态

isolation /ˌaɪsəˈleɪʃn/ *n*. separation, putting or keeping apart from others 隔离

dissociation /dɪˌsəʊsɪˈeɪʃn/, /dɪˌsəʊʃɪˈeɪʃn/ *n*. separation (people or things) in one's thoughts or feelings（在思想或感情方面）将（人或事物）分开

depletion /dɪˈpliːʃn/ *n*. depleting or being depleted 消耗；消减

essence /ˈesns/ *n*. that which makes a thing what it is; most important or indispensable quality of sth. 本质；精髓；要素；（中医上指）精气

wax /wæks/ *n*. & *vi*. increase in power, strength, importance, etc. 增加；增长

---

①   "being restricted" and "restricting"："克我"和"我克"。
②   wood subjugating earth：木乘土。
③   Counter-restriction refers to the idea of the strong one bullying the weak：相侮，从字面上讲就是依强欺弱。
④   wood counter-restricting metal：木侮金。

wane /weɪn/ *n. & vi.* decrease in power, strength, importance, etc. 衰退

peripherally /pəˈrɪfərəlɪ/ *adv.* in or at or near a periphery or according to a peripheral role or function or relationship 周边地；外围地；次要地

subjugation /ˌsʌbdʒuˈɡeɪʃn/ *n.* forced submission to control by others 征服；镇压；克制

FOLLOW-UP ACTIVITIES

Task one   Comprehension Check

1. Questions for Discussion

1) Please list adjectives as many as possible to describe female qualities and male qualities.

2) How do you understand the statement of "extreme *yin* turns into *yang* and extreme *yang* into *yin*"?

3) Why is the liver attributed to wood?

4) Discuss the application of *yin-yang* theory in TCM.

5) Discuss the application of five element theory in TCM?

2. Chart Completion

INTRODUCTION: (para. 1)

The philosophical concepts of traditional Chinese medicine reflect a 1) _____ concept of materialism and dialectics and have played an active role in promoting the development of 2) _____ in China. In the ancient times, these philosophical concepts were applied to the field of medicine and greatly influenced the 3) _____ of TCM.

Concept of *Yin* and *Yang* of TCM: (para. 2 – 6)

Yin and *yang* are the summary of 4) _____ of two opposite aspects of interrelated things or phenomena in nature. *Yin* and *yang* 5) _____ each other. *Yin* and *yang* 6) _____ each other. *Yin* and *yang* 7) _____ each other. *Yin* and *yang* 8) _____ each other.

Concept of Five Elements of TCM: (para. 7 – 14)

The five elements refer to wood, fire, earth, metal and water as well as their 9) _____ in the natural world. Wood is characterized by 10) _____. Fire is characterized by 11) _____. Earth is characterized by 12) _____. Metal is characterized by changing. Water is characterized by 13) _____.

The movement of the five elements is mainly characterized by 14) _____, and mutual interaction between mother and child.

Summary: (para. 15)

The philosophical concepts of *yin-yang* and five elements permeate through all aspects of the theoretical system of TCM. When applied into TCM, they serve to explain the organic structure, 15) _____ of the human body, and in addition, guide clinical diagnosis and treatment.

Task Two　Vocabulary

1. Directions: Complete the following phrases respectively according to its corresponding meaning or equivalent in Chinese within the brackets.

1) _____（属性的）summarization

2) _____（相互关联的）things or phenomena

3) _____（相反的）side

4) _____（双重的）aspect

5) brightness and_____（暗）

6) _____（病态的）condition

7) ascending and _____（下降）

8) _____（对立）between *yin* and *yang*

9) mutual _____（补充）

10) opposition and_____（制约）

11) dynamic_____（平衡）

12) _____（互根互用）between *yin* and *yang*

13) _____（离绝）of *yin* and *yang*

14) _____（消长）between *yin* and *yang*

15) _____（相互转化）between *yin* and *yang*

16) *yin* _____（证）

17) _____（不断的）motion

18) _____（生理的）function

19) clinical diagnosis and _____（治疗）

20) cultivation and _____（稿）

21) supporting and _____（受纳）

22) _____（净化）and descending

23) _____（滋润）and downward flowing

24) wood _____（生）fire

25) earth_____（克）water

26) wood _____（乘）earth

27) wood _____（侮）metal

28) _____（病理的）change

29) _____（消耗）of essence

30) primitive_____（概念）

2. Match the following words with their proper meanings.

Column I	Column II
1) attribute	a.　that depend on each other; consisting of parts that depend on each other
2) connotation	b.　to exist together in the same place or at the same time, especially in a peaceful way

continued

Column I	Column II
3) reverse	c. a quality or feature of sb./sth.
4) dimness	d. to spread to every part of an object or a place
5) contradiction	e. an idea suggested by a word in addition to its main meaning
6) quiescence	f. mutual or reciprocal relation or relatedness
7) interdependent	g. to change sth. completely so that it is the opposite of what it was before
8) coexist	h. a lack of agreement between facts, opinions, actions, etc.
9) counterpart	i. constrict or bind or draw together
10) permeate	j. a mutual or reciprocal action; interacting
11) interrelation	k. the state of being poorly illuminated
12) astringe	l. using an idea or a statement to prove sth. which is then used to prove the idea or statement at the beginning
13) interaction	m. a person or thing that has the same position or function as sb./sth. else in a different place or situation
14) circular	n. to harm sb. who is weaker than you, or make use of them in a dishonest way to get what you want
15) prey	o. the state or quality of being quiescent

3. Fill in the blanks with the words from the box and change the form when necessary.

circular	counterpart	deplete	dimness	contradiction
quiescence	interaction	prey	permeate	interrelation
attribute	coexist	connotation	reverse	complementation

1) The committee refused to _____ blame without further information.

2) This study showed without question that collaboration is grounded in human _____ and relationships.

3) "Most cells in the immune system are in a state of _____ , not running around with their hair on fire all the time," he said.

4) The buildings, with a _____ shape and a flat roof, were made of mud and stone.

5) The word "professional" has _____ of skill and excellence.

6) But according to data from the United Nations, US doctors write five and a half times more prescriptions for opioids (阿片类药物) than do their _____ in France, and eight times more than do physicians in Italy.

7) The study, published in Psychological Science, went one step further: it suggested that personality and happiness do not merely _____ , but that in fact innate personality traits cause happiness.

8) On top of their incandescent (十分明亮的) beauty, fireflies are considered important in the

ecosystem, _____ upon creatures such as slugs (蛞蝓) and snails.

9) And if normal cells are found to be removed by senescent (衰老的) cells in aged tissues, this _____ might contribute directly to tissue degeneration .

10) Ethanol (乙醇) has severe injury effect in the development of cerebrum (大脑), nevertheless, the mechanism of action is still _____ .

11) But it is the _____ among these four elements that is the most novel and distinctive aspect of McLean's account.

12) And in a world increasingly _____ by distractions — a major contributor to traffic accidents — any insights into how the brain works should get our attention.

13) By learning more about the roles of RNA (核糖核酸) in cardiovascular disease, researchers hope to harness the molecules to prevent and even _____ key steps in the process.

14) His public speeches are in direct _____ to his personal lifestyle.

15) They are _____ rather than contradictory, but they differ in their aims.

Task Three   Translation

1. Translate the following medical expressions into English

1) 哲学概念	2) 阴阳转化
3) 阴平阳秘	4) 寒极生热
5) 相互消长	6) 相互制约
7) 相互依存	8) 相反相成
9) 病理变化	10) 有机结构
11) 五行学说	12) 生我、我生
13) 木曰曲直	14) 土爱稼穑
15) 相乘相侮	16) 火曰炎上
17) 金曰从革	18) 水曰润下
19) 土虚木乘	20) 母病及子

2. Translate the following sentences into Chinese or English

1) *Yin* and *yang* are the summary of the attributes of two opposite aspects of interrelated things or phenomena in nature.

2) Water and fire are the symbols of *yin* and *yang*.

3) Each of the five elements is marked by such relations as "being generated" and "generating".

4) In this circular order, each of the five elements is marked by "being restricted" and "restricting".

5) It is a morbid condition in which one element fails to restrict the other in the regular order, but is restricted by the other in the reverse order.

6) 凡具有温热、升腾作用的事物,均归属于火。(attributed to)

7) 相生指这一事物对另一事物具有促进、助长和资生的作用。(bring forth)

8) 换句话说,没有功能活动,物质的新陈代谢就无法进行;没有必要的物质,功能活动也就无从发

挥。(be carried out)

9) 正是通过这种对立和制约,才能够建立动态平衡。(it is just through ...)

10) 五行学说认为,宇宙中所有的现象在本质上都与木、火、土、金、水相对应,这些元素处于不断运动和变化的状态。(correspond to)

3. Translate the following passage into English

　　阴阳五行学说对后来古代唯物主义哲学有着深远的影响,在长期医疗实践的基础上,将阴阳五行学说广泛地运用于医学领域,用以说明人类生命起源、生理现象、病理变化,指导着临床的诊断和防治,成为中医理论的重要组成部分,对中医学理论体系的形成和发展,起着极为深刻的影响。

 Text B

Taiji: A Great Myth

1　The basic pattern of the **interaction** of *yin* and *yang* in traditional Chinese medicine is best illustrated by the Taiji Circle.

2　Taiji is often translated as "Supreme Ultimate". This symbol **depicts** a cycle in time and space. Beginning **arbitrarily** with the birth of *yin* (the narrowest portion of the dark half of the circle), the course of the cycle follows its growth, with the **concomitant** decrease of *yang*, to its greatest fullness. At its height, when it seems to have **obliterated** *yang*, *yin* contains seeds of both *yang* and its obliteration. From this seed (the small light-colored dot in the middle of the largest area of darkness, known as the "mother *yang*"), *yang* takes root and begins its own cycle of growth. This aspect implies that there is always *yin* within *yang* and *yang* within *yin* in the real world.

3　To illustrate this process, let's consider "weakness" as an example of *yin*, and "strength" as an example of *yang*. We can see how a person's weakness might steadily increase, allowing it to do less and less until the weakness is so **debilitating** that it "commands" the aid of caretakers; thus, this very weakness actually overpowers or enlists the strength of others. *Yin* has become *yang*.

4　In the same manner, physical strength may grow, its exuberance leading it to more and more expression, until it cannot stop itself. Then, by its mere appearance, the slightest weakness can stimulate it to act (e.g., like a vulnerable kid standing next to a bully). And strength, having lost control of itself, finds itself

interaction /ˌɪntərˈækʃn/　*n*. 相互作用,相互影响;交流

depict /dɪˈpɪkt/　*v*. 描写;描述;刻画

arbitrarily /ˌɑːbɪˈtrerəlɪ/　*adv*. 任意地,随意地

concomitant /kənˈkɒmɪtənt/ *adj*.(尤指相关联的或有因果关系的事)同时发生的,伴随的

obliterate /əˈblɪtəreɪt/　*v*. 毁掉;覆盖;清除

debilitating /dɪˈbɪlɪteɪtɪŋ/ *adj*. 使衰弱的

overpowered by weakness. *Yang* has become *yin*. The roles have reversed. This is one example of how the cycle of mutual growth and displacement of *yin* and *yang* works in the Taiji.

5　The weakening of one side of the equation necessarily leads to the strengthening of the other, and the **alternation** of *yin* and *yang* perpetuates itself. This alternation produces undifferentiated *qi*, or "energy" in the broadest sense of the word, similar to the alternation of positive and negative that produce electricity in an electric motor. And the behavior of *qi* itself follows the rules of the Taiji in ever smallest **microcosms** — like eddies in the flow of a great river — ultimately producing and forming all the phenomena of the universe.

6　In other words, matter is just the tendency of energy — *qi* — to behave in particular ways. It can be described as a function of the behavior of its constituent *yin* and *yang*.

7　The cycle of these two factors can be seen in the alternation of day and night, in the seasons of the year, in the rise and fall of empires and dynasties, in human life and in the body itself.

8　All phenomena in the world may be seen as part of this never-ending cycle of change and transformation. Nothing comes into being and nothing ceases to be; forms and appearances change, but the fact of change is constant, and *qi*, is the substance of everything.

9　The arbitrariness of this description of the universe is evident and acknowledged. It is recognized in modern western physics that there is no real or definable distinction between one **atom** and another, and by extention, one thing and another. As in physics, everything can be seen as a function of energy, and therefore in reality is stripped of its collective characteristics; so in Taiji theory, the universe is really Wuji.

10　Wu means "without" or "no". Ji may be translated as extreme, very, ultimate, but its basic meaning is "pole", as North Pole or South Pole. It implies an extreme, but it is impossible to divorce this extreme from its opposite extreme, and from the continuum that they define. Consider one end a stick. Without the stick, there can be no end. And without the other end, there can also be no stick. Thus, each end implies the other, as well as the stick that they both define.

11　Wuji means an absence of any such pole. In other words,

---

alternation /ˌɔːltəˈneɪʃn/　*n.* 交替,轮流,间隔

microcosm /ˈmaɪkrəʊkɒzəm/ *n.* 微观世界；小宇宙；作为宇宙缩影的人

atom /ˈætəm/ *n.* 原子

there is no **dichotomy** to provide a basis for measurement, definition, or existence. Wuji is essentially viewed as chaos, and chaos is seen as the underlying reality of the world.

dichotomy /daɪˈkɒtəmɪ/ *n*. 二分法;两分;分裂

12   The *Dao De Jing* (Chapter 42) states that "from one comes two, from two comes three, and from three comes all". When you declare the existence of a "thing", then within chaos there is a dichotomy — there is "that thing" on the one hand, and there is "whatever is not that thing" on the other. Once you allow a dichotomy, there are at least three things — one end of the dichotomy, the other end of the dichotomy, and the whole of the system. And once this definition of the central dichotomy and the whole system has been made, it can be **elaborated** infinitely. Making the first distinction logically **entails** every phenomenon that can be distinguished. In this sense, Wuji might be understood as "no distinction," and Taiji as "first distinction".

elaborate /ɪˈlæb(ə)rət/ *v*. 详尽阐述;详细描述
entail /ɪnˈteɪl/ *v*. 牵涉;需要;使必要

13   As the first distinction is arbitrary, the dichotomy distinguished may be arbitrarily defined. In the Chinese tradition "light and shade" (*yang* and *yin*) form the Taiji, mutually defining each other, and so, within chaos, mutually create each other. Light, in Western physics is energy, movement and change; shade in contrast is stability, stillness, and form. There is no change unless there are forms that change, and there is no form that has not become, i.e., changed into, its form. But once light and shade begin transforming, the whole world can exist. The cycle of change and transformation has begun, and from this the three main currents of *yin* and three main currents of *yang* are evident.
(948 words)

Notes:

1. The basic pattern of interaction of *yin* and *yang* in traditional Chinese medicine is best illustrated by the Taiji Circle. 太极图最能说明中医阴阳交互作用的基本模式。

2. alternation of *yin* and *yang* 阴阳交替

3. And the behavior of *qi* itself follows the rules of the Taiji in ever smallest microcosms — like eddies in the flow of a great river — ultimately producing and forming all the phenomena of the universe. 在任何最小的微观世界中,气本身的行为遵循着太极的规则——就像一条大河中的漩涡——最终产生和形成了宇宙的所有现象。

4. Ji may be translated as extreme, very, ultimate, but its basic meaning is "pole", as in North Pole or South Pole."极"可以翻译为"极端的""极""终极的",但它的基本意思是"极点",如北极或南极。

5. The *Dao De Jing* (Chapter 42) states that "from one comes two, from two comes three, and

from three comes all". 《道德经》(42 章) 曰: "一生二, 二生三, 三生万物。"

Task One   Reading Comprehension

1. Taiji Circle symbolizes _____ .

   A. the basic interaction between *yin* and *yang*   B. the decline of *yin* and *yang*

   C. the growth of *yin*   D. the development of *yang*

2. The conception of Taiji implies that _____ .

   A. *yin* and *yang* are always opposing each other

   B. there is always *yin* within *yang* and *yang* within *yin*

   C. there is always *yin* within *yang* but no *yang* within *yin*

   D. *yin* and *yang* are always divorcing from each other

3. According to the passage, all the following elements are the examples of the cycle of *yin* and *yang* EXCEPT _____ .

   A. the alternation of day and night   B. the seasons in a year

   C. family and home   D. human life and the body itself

4. According to the passage, Ji means _____ .

   A. no   B. cycle   C. chaos   D. pole

5. In the sentence "As the first distinction is arbitrary", the word "distinction" means _____ .

   A. instinct   B. intuitive   C. difference   D. categorization

Task Two   Vocabulary

1. **Directions: Complete the following phrases respectively according to its corresponding meaning or equivalent in Chinese within the brackets.**

1) basic _____ (模式)   2) _____ (至高的) ultimate

3) _____ (交互作用) of *yin* and *yang*   4) _____ (伴随的) decrease

5) _____ (稳定地) increase   6) _____ (身体的) strength

7) _____ (只不过) appearance   8) mutual _____ (取代)

9) positive and _____ (消极的)   10) smallest _____ (微观世界)

11) _____ (现象) of the universe   12) _____ (趋势) of energy

13) _____ (永无止境的) cycle   14) _____ (交替) of *yin* and *yang*

15) _____ (公认的) description   16) definable _____ (区别)

17) _____ (共同的) characteristics   18) _____ (存在) of a "thing"

19) central _____ (二分法)   20) _____ (任意的) distinction

2. **Fill in the blanks with the words from the box and change the form when necessary.**

overpower	enlist	alternation	stimulate	equation
ultimate	illustrate	undifferentiated	elaborate	never-ending
strip	underlying	stability	continuum	transformation

1）The stress of life seems to have _____ many of their passion and excitement.

2）With a crucial vote on health care expected Tuesday in the Senate（参议院）Finance Committee, the president sought to _____ medical professionals in the cause.

3）His lecture was _____ with slides taken during the expedition.

4）Police finally managed to _____ the gunman.

5）Would you like to learn some lessons in life from the _____ minimalist（简约主义者）?

6）The way in which we work has undergone a complete _____ in the past decade.

7）It is impossible to say at what point along the _____ a dialect becomes a separate language.

8）This is in large part because of our biological predilection（偏爱）for homeostasis（体内平衡）, or physiological _____ , which prompts our bodies to regain any weight that we lose and, in theory, lose any weight that we gain.

9）Older people and those with _____ health problems are more likely to suffer.

10）If the eastern side falls apart, then the entire _____ will change.

11）All plants maintain this dual life cycle, called "the _____ of generations".

12）Four were taken to a hospital in Washington state, while Scott Pauley, a CDC（疾控中心）spokesman, wouldn't _____ on where the others were taken.

13）Exposure to unfamiliar speech sounds is initially registered by the brain as _____ neural activity.

14）The women were given fertility drugs to _____ the ovaries（卵巢）.

15）Children ask a seemingly _____ stream of questions from an early age.

Task Three   Writing

Please rewrite the text in a form of abstract（about 150 words）

Terminology

Basic Terminology of TCM Philosophical Concepts

Terminology	WHO	WFCMS
阴阳	*yin* and *yang*	*yin* and *yang*；*yin-yang*
阴阳转化	*yin-yang* conversion	*yin-yang* conversion
阴阳偏盛	abnormal exuberance of *yin* or *yang*	abnormal exuberance of *yin* or *yang*
阴阳两虚证	pattern/syndrome of dual deficiency of *yin* and *yang*	syndrome/pattern of both *yin* and *yang* deficiency
阴阳辨证	*yin-yang* pattern identification/syndrome differentiation	*yin-yang* syndrome differentiation/pattern identification
阴阳毒	*yin* toxin(阴毒)；*yang* toxin(阳毒)	*yin* and *yang* toxin
阴阳否隔	无	stagnation of *yin* and *yang*

continued

Terminology	WHO	WFCMS
阴阳乖戾	无	*yin-yang* imbalance
阴阳互不相抱	无	divorce of *yin* and *yang*
阴阳互根	mutual rooting of *yin* and *yang*	mutual rooting of *yin* and *yang*
阴阳交	无	*yin-yang* interlocking
阴阳交感	无	interaction of *yin* and *yang*
阴阳俱虚	无	deficiency of dual *yin* and *yang*
阴阳离决，精气乃绝	无	If *yin* and *yang* separate from each other, essential *qi* will be exhausted.
阴阳偏衰	abnormal debilitation of *yin* or *yang*	abnormal debilitation of *yin* or *yang*
阴阳平衡	*yin-yang* balance	*yin-yang* balance
阴阳气并竭	无	exhaustion of *yang* and *yin*
阴阳胜复	无	alternative preponderance of *yin* and *yang*
阴阳失调	*yin-yang* disharmony	*yin-yang* disharmony
阴阳调和	*yin-yang* harmony	*yin-yang* harmony
阴阳消长	waxing and waning of *yin* and *yang*	waning and waxing of *yin* and *yang*
阴阳自和	spontaneous harmonization of *yin* and *yang*	spontaneous harmonization of *yin* and *yang*
阴中之阳	*yang* within *yin*	*yang* within *yin*
阴中之阴	*yin* within *yin*	*yin* within *yin*
五行学说	five phase theory	five-element/phase theory
五行相乘	overwhelming(相乘)	over-restriction among five elements/phases
五行相克	restraining(相克)	restriction among five elements/phases
五行相生	engendering(相生)	generation of five elements/phases
五行相侮	mutual inhibition(相恶)	counter-restriction among five elements/phases

本书配套数字教学资源

微信扫描二维码，加入中医英语
读者交流圈，获取配套教学视
频、学习课件、课后习题和沟通交
流平台等板块内容，夯实基础知识

The five viscera appear as one body
The viscera and bowels are mutually connected
五脏一体 脏腑相合①

Unit 3 Theory of Visceral Manifestation

Warming-up

Before you listen(Watch)

In this section you will hear a short passage about "*Zang Fu*". The following words and phrases may be of help.

acupuncturist /ˈækjʊˌpʌŋktʃərɪst/	*n.*	针灸师
herbalist /ˈhɜː(r)bəlɪst/	*n.*	草药医生;草药专家
oriental /ˌɔːrɪˈentəl/	*a.*	东方的
disharmony /ˈdɪsˈhɑː(r)mənɪ/	*n.*	不调和
progression /prəˈgreʃən/	*n.*	前进;进展
recurrence /rɪˈkʌrəns/	*n.*	复发;反复
transformer /trænsˈfɔː(r)mə(r)/	*n.*	促使改变的人或物
bioenergetics /ˈbaɪəʊˌenə(r)ˈdʒetɪks/	*n.*	生物能学
congenital /kənˈdʒenɪtəl/	*a.*	先天的
spleen /spliːn/	*n.*	脾
pancreas /ˈpæŋkrɪəs/	*n.*	胰
nourish /ˈnʌrɪʃ/	*v.*	养育;滋养
moisten /ˈmɔɪsən/	*v.*	使变得潮湿;变得湿润
lubricate /ˈluːbrɪkeɪt/	*v.*	使润滑
spinal /ˈspaɪnəl/	*a.*	脊柱的;脊髓的
synovial /saɪˈnəʊvɪəl/	*a.*	滑液的

---

① *Statements of Facts in Traditional Chinese Medicine*, Bob Flaws 著。

While you listen(Watch)

Listen to the passage carefully and fill in each of the blanks marked from 1) to 10) according to what you have heard.

Welcome to *American Dragon Presents*: Chinese Medicine in America. I'm a licensed acupuncturist and herbalist and a professor of oriental medicine. In this episode, we begin to discuss the 1) _____ organs or *zang fu*, in order to understand the human body, discover the imbalances that result in 2) _____, predict the progression of imbalance, and prevent recurrence. The Chinese organs are vastly different from the western organs. The *zang fu* are energy transformers or *qi* transformers in a bioenergetic 3) _____. And what they do relates to their *qi* transformation functions.

Qi is the vital energetic force that gives life to all things. There are three sources of *qi*. The first source of *qi* is congenital *qi*, stored in the kidneys. It can perform 4) _____ functions within the body. The next source of *qi* is called clean air *qi*. It is received by the lungs and transformed into *qi* that 5) _____ different functions. And the last source of *qi* is food and drink, which is received by the stomach, processed and sent to the spleen and pancreas for transformation. The organs also transform 6) _____ or *qi* patterns into physical manifestations. We can trace the source of the imbalance, predict potential problems, treat them, and prevent them from occurring. Physical problems manifest when the energetic source is out of balance.

The five substances are also known as the five treasures, including *qi*, *jing*, blood, *shen* and body fluids. *Qi* is the 7) _____ substance in the universe. *Jing* is a specialized form of *qi* that contains the blueprint for our life on earth. Blood is another specialized type of *qi* that 8) _____ and moistens the cells. *Shen* is another very special form of *qi* which is the decision maker and resides in the heart. Body fluids are another specific form of *qi* which cool, moisten and lubricate the body. There are thin fluids called *jin*, such as tears and 9) _____. And there are thick fluids, like spinal or synovial fluid called *ye*.

My hope is that by understanding this system, you will have new 10) _____ about how the human body functions and how you can live a healthy, happy life.

After you listen(Watch)

Please discuss with your partner the following questions and give your presentation to the class.

1) What is oriental medicine? Is it the same as Chinese medicine?
2) Why are the Chinese organs vastly different from the western organs?
3) How can physical problems be prevented from occurring?
4) Can you describe *shen* in your own words?

Reading

 Text A

BEFORE CLASS

1. Quest for Definition

Directions: Explore online the definitions of the following terms from Text A and prepare a unique one-minute oral presentation for your class.

1) visceral manifestation
2) extraordinary *fu*-organs
3) organic holism
4) "The liver opens into the eyes."
5) fullness and solidity (of the *zang-fu* organs)
6) "Viscera inside the body must manifest themselves externally."

2. Text-based Activities

Directions: Read carefully the part of Text A that corresponds to your task, and then prepare a unique one-minute oral presentation in a unique way for class.

PERFORMANCE IN CLASS

Your Task

1) How can the phrase "*zang xiang*" be interpreted?

2) What are the physiological functions and functional characteristics of *zang*-organs and *fu*-organs respectively?

3) What is an extraordinary *fu*-organ?

4) What is the significance to differentiate *zang*-organs from *fu*-organs in clinical practice?

5) On what basis has the theory of visceral manifestation been developed?

The Theory of Visceral Manifestation

1　The phrase visceral manifestation or *zang xiang* in Chinese first appeared in the *Chapter of Six Sections of Discussion on Visceral Manifestation* in *Su Wen* (*Basic Questions*)①. According to the

---

①　*Chapter of Six Sections of Discussion on Visceral Manifestation* in *Su Wen* (*Plain Questions*)：《素问·六节藏象论篇》。

explanations in some Chinese medical classics, "*zang*" refers to the interior organs which are stored inside the body, and "*xiang*" refers to exterior manifestations of physiological functions and pathological changes of internal organs. In the *Lei Jing* (*Canon of Classification*)[1] compiled by Zhang Jingyue in 1624 CE, for example, it was recorded that "*xiang* means image". The viscera are contained inside the body and their images are manifested outward. For this reason, it is called "visceral manifestation"[2]. And *zang xiang* is sometimes translated as "viscera and their manifestations".

2   The theory of visceral manifestation studies the physiological functions and pathological changes of viscera and their corresponding relationships. It plays an important role in building the theoretical system of TCM and is significant for expounding the physiology and pathology of the human body and for guiding clinical practice.

3   Viscera, basis for the theory of visceral manifestation, is a collective term of the internal organs which, according to their physiological functions, can be classified into three major categories: the five *zang*-organs, including the heart, liver, spleen, lung and kidney; the six *fu*-organs, including the gallbladder, stomach, small intestine, large intestine, bladder and triple energizers; and the extraordinary *fu*-organs, including the brain, marrow, bone, vessel, gallbladder and uterus.

4   The common physiological function of the five *zang*-organs is to transform and store essence; while that of the six fu-organs is to receive, transport and transform water and food. The extraordinary *fu*-organs, as a type of *fu*-organs, differing from the six *fu*-organs in shape and physiological function, are relatively hermetic organs and do not contact with water and food directly. So in the *Chapter of Special Discussion on Five Zang-organs* in *Su Wen*, it was described that "the so-called five *zang*-organs refer to the organs that only store essence but not excrete it; that is the reason why they can be full but not solid. The six *fu*-organs are in charge of transporting and transforming food, so they can be solid but not full. The reason is that the stomach becomes full and the intestines remain empty when food is taken into the stomach through the mouth; the intestines become solid and the stomach gets empty when food is transported downward. That is what to be full but not to be solid and to be solid but not to be full means."[3]

5   The above mentioned fullness and solidity actually refer to the characteristics of essence and food. Wang Bing[4] said, "Essence is characterized by fullness and food by solidness. Since the five *zang*-organs only store essence, they can just be full, but not solid; the function of the six *fu*-organs is to receive food but not to store essence, so they only can be solid but not full[5]."

---

①   *Lei Jing* (*Canon of Classification*):《类经》。

②   "*xiang* means image". The viscera are contained inside the body and their images are manifested outwardly. For this reason, it is called "visceral manifestation":"象,形象也。"藏居于内,形见于外,故曰"藏象"。

③   That is what to be full but not to be solid and to be solid but not to be full means:"故曰,实而不满,满而不实也。"

④   Wang Bing：王冰。

⑤   Essence is characterized by fullness and food by solidness. Since the five *zang*-organs only store essence, they can just be full, but not solid; the function of the six *fu*-organs is to receive food but not to store essence, so they only can be solid but not full:精气为满,水谷为实。五脏但藏精气,故满而不实;六腑则不藏精气,但受水谷,故实而不能满也。

6   The significance for differentiating between the *zang*-organs and the *fu*-organs is not only for explaining their physiological functions, but also for guiding clinical practice. For instance, the disorders of *zang*-organs are mostly of deficiency type; while the disorders of *fu*-organs are mainly of excess type. The related *fu*-organ can be **purged** for the treatment of the excess type of *zang*-organ disorders, and the related *zang*-organ can be nourished for the treatment of the deficiency type of *fu*-organ disorders. These therapeutic principles are still of great significance① for guiding clinical practice even today.

7   The theory of visceral manifestation advanced on the basis of the development of the following three aspects.

8   (1) The knowledge of anatomy accumulated in ancient times. In the *Ling Shu* (*The Spiritual Pivot*), for instance, it says, "The eight-*chi* human body may be measured on the surface. After death, the body may be **dissected** and the **texture** of the *zang*-organs, the size of the *fu*-organs, the capacity of the intestines, the length of the **vessels**, the condition of the blood can also be observed..."From a basic anatomic point of view, understanding the human body laid a solid foundation for the theory of visceral manifestation in **morphology**.

9   (2) The long-term observation of the human physiological functions and pathological changes. For example, since catching a cold may produce such symptoms as **stuffy** nose, running nose and cough, the ancient people gradually came to realize that there was a close relationship between the skin and hair with the nose and lung.

10   (3) The repeated medical practice in which certain physiological functions were disproved and analyzed in the light of pathological phenomena and **curative** effect. For example, because eye disorders were mostly cured by treating the liver, the ancient people eventually reached the conclusion that "the liver opens into the eyes".

11   The theory of visceral manifestation is mainly characterized by the concept of organic holism. According to this theory, the *zang*-organs pertain to *yin* and the *fu*-organs to *yang*. Each *zang*-organ is internally and externally related to a certain *fu*-organ. For example, the heart is internally and externally related to the small intestine, the lung to the large intestine, the spleen to the stomach, the liver to the gallbladder, the kidney to the bladder and the **pericardium** to the triple energizers. These internal and external relations are **deduced** on the basis of the interconnection between meridians.

12   Physiological functions are closely related to mental and emotional activities. Spirit, consciousness and thinking reflect the functions of the brain, which was already mentioned in *Nei Jing* (*The Internal Classic*). However, the theory of visceral manifestation holds that spirit, consciousness and thinking are also closely related to the physiological functions of the five *zang*-organs. Since the physiological functions of the five *zang*-organs control the whole body, the brain also depends on the five *zang*-organs to perform its physiological functions. So the balance of the five *zang*-organs' physiological functions is the key to internal environment of the human body.

---

①   of great significance: ……具有重要意义。

13 The above analysis shows that the theory of visceral manifestation, though based on ancient anatomy, was established mainly by means of observation according to the idea that "viscera inside the body must manifest themselves externally①." Therefore, the result of the observation and analysis was inevitably beyond the viscera in human anatomy. From this, TCM has developed such a unique system for physiology and pathology.

14 As a result, the heart, lung, spleen, liver and kidney in the theory of visceral manifestation differ greatly in physiology and pathology from the corresponding organs in the modern human anatomy. In fact, the physiological function of one internal organ in the theory of visceral manifestation may include that of several internal organs in the modern human anatomy. Similarly, the physiological function of one organ in the modern human anatomy may be involved in that of several organs in the theory of visceral manifestation. This is due to the fact that the viscera in the theory of visceral manifestation is not only a simple anatomical concept, but also a concept that generalizes the physiology and pathology of a certain system. (1,201 words)

New Words and Expressions

viscera /ˈvɪsərə/ *n*. the large inside organs of the body, such as the heart, lungs, stomach, etc. 内脏;脏腑

gallbladder /ˈɡɔːlˌblædə/ *n*. the organ in your body in which bile stored 胆囊

energizer /ˈenədʒaɪzə/ *n*. someone who imparts energy and vitality and spirit to other people; a device that supplies electrical energy 激发器;增能器;(在中医上)焦

marrow /ˈmærəʊ/ *n*. the soft fatty substance in the hollow centre of bones 骨髓

vessel /ˈvesl/ *n*. a tubular structure that transports such body fluids as blood and lymph 脉管

uterus /ˈjuːtərəs/ *n*. womb 子宫

transform /trænsˈfɔːm/ *v*. to completely change the appearance, form, or character of something or someone, especially in a way that improves it 使改变;转换

excrete /ɪkˈskriːt/ *vt*. eliminate from the body 排泄;排出

purge /pɜːdʒ/ *v*. clear waste matter from (the bowels) 使通便;(在中医上)泻

dissect /dɪˈsekt, daɪˈsekt/ *v*. to cut up the body of a dead animal or person in order to study it 解剖

texture /ˈtekstʃə(r)/ *n*. the way a surface or material feels when you touch it, especially how smooth or rough it is 质地

morphology /mɔːˈfɒlədʒɪ/ *n*. the structure or formation of an object or system 结构;形态

stuffy /ˈstʌfɪ/ *adj*. a room or building that is stuffy does not have enough fresh air in it 不通气的;窒息的

curative /ˈkjʊərətɪv/ *adj*. able to, or intended to cure illness 治疗的;治愈的

pericardium /ˌperɪˈkɑːdɪəm/ *n*. a double-layered serous membrane that surrounds the heart 心包

deduce /dɪˈdjuːs/ *vt*. to use the knowledge and information you have in order to understand something or form an opinion about it 推论;演绎

---

① viscera inside the body must manifest themselves externally：有诸内,必形诸外。

FOLLOW-UP ACTIVITIES

Task one   Comprehension Check

1. **Questions for Discussion**

1) How do the *zang-fu* organs in the theory of visceral manifestation differ from those in Western medicine? Can you give an example?

2) How do you understand the "harmony between the heart and kidney"?

3) Can you explain how the *zang-fu* organs are involved in the water/fluid transmission and excretion according to TCM theory?

4) In TCM theory, the spleen could be damaged by emotional factors like over-thinking. Is there any evidence of the causal relationship between emotional disorder and gastrointestinal diseases in Western medicine?

2. **Chart Completion**

INTRODUCTION: (para. 1 - 2)

Initially appearing in *Su Wen*, the phrase of visceral manifestation or *zang xiang* refers to a unique theoretical system in TCM. In the theory of *zang xiang*, "*zang*" refers to 1) _____ _____ which are contained inside the body and "*xiang*" refers to 2) _____ of physiological functions and pathological changes of internal organs. Such a theory is significant for both explicating the 3) _____ of the human body and guiding 4) _____ .

CLASSIFICATION OF THE VISCERA, AND THEIR PHYSIOLOGICAL AND CLINICAL FUNCTIONS: (para. 3 - 6)

In the theory of visceral manifestation, viscera, as a collective term of internal organs, is further divided into three groups according to their physiological functions, namely, the five *zang*-organs, including 5) _____ , the six *fu*-organs, including 6) _____ , and the extraordinary *fu*-organs, including 7) ____ _____ .

The significance of such a classification is twofold. On one hand, it provides the framework for the explanation of the physiological functions of the internal organs. The physiological functions of the five *zang*-organs is to 8) _____ essence, while the six *fu*-organs work to 9) _____ water and food. That is why in *Su Wen*, *zang*-organs are described as being 10) _____ , and *fu*-organs as being 11) _____ . The extraordinary *fu*-organs differ from the *fu*-organs in 12) _____ _____ . The visceral manifestation also serves as the evidence for choosing the suitable therapeutic principle in clinical practice. Generally, the disorders of *zang*-organs are mostly of 13) _____ type, which can be treated by 14) _____ ; while the disorders of the *fu*-organs are mostly of 15) _____ type, which is usually treated by

16) _____ .

THEORETICAL BASIS: (para. 7 – 10)

The theory of visceral manifestation advanced on the basis of the development of the following three aspects, namely, the 17) _____ accumulated in ancient times, the long-term observation of the human 18) _____ _____ , and the repeated medical practice based on 19) _____ .

MORE THAN A SIMPLE ANATOMICAL CONCEPT: (para. 11 – 14)

The theory of visceral manifestation is mainly characterized by the concept of 20) _____ _____ , which is manifested as internal-external relation between the *zang-fu* organs on the basis of 21) _____ , as well as close relationship between physiological functions of internal organs and 22) _____ .

Therefore, such a theory, though based on ancient anatomy, is more than a simple anatomical concept, but a concept that 23) _____ the physiological functions and pathological changes of a certain system.

Task Two Vocabulary

1. **Directions: Complete the following phrases respectively according to its corresponding meaning or equivalent in Chinese within the brackets.**

1) _____(外在的) manifestations

2) _____(解剖) human body

3) _____(生理的) functions

4) _____(整体性的) approach of healing

5) _____(实) pattern

6) _____(精神的) illness

7) _____(临床的) practice

8) _____(情绪的) turbulence

9) _____(器质性的) diseases

10) disorders of _____(意识)

11) _____ manifestation(藏象)

12) _____(解剖的) variation

13) _____(虚) pattern

14) _____(形态学的) analysis

15) the knowledge of _____(解剖)

16) _____(泻) heart fire

17) _____(治疗的) principle

18) _____(滋养) kidney *yin*

19) _____(内在的) environment of the human body

20) _____（保持）of *yin-yang* balance

21) _____（相互联结）between meridians

22) _____（区分）between *zang*-organs and *fu*-organs

23) concrete _____（基础）

24) skin _____（纹理）

25) _____（反驳）an argument

26) coronary _____（动脉）

27) _____（治疗的;有效的）effect

28) transporting and _____（消化;转化）

29) store _____（精）

30) _____（推断）relations

2. Match the following words with their proper meanings.

Column I	Column II
1) physiological	a. to keep a person, an animal or a plant alive and healthy with food, etc.
2) hermetic	b. connected with or happening in the mind; involving the process of thinking
3) corresponding	c. the act of making a state or situation continue
4) mental	d. to explain something by talking about it in detail
5) pathological	e. connected with the scientific study of the normal functions of living things
6) capacity	f. done or shared by all members of a group of people; involving a whole group or society
7) expound	g. to apply a theory, idea, etc. to a wider group or situation than the original one
8) generalize	h. tightly closed so that no air can escape or enter
9) collective	i. caused by, or connected with, disease or illness
10) holism	j. to show that something is wrong or false
11) nourish	k. an event, action or thing that is a sign that something exists or is happening
12) disprove	l. the idea that the whole of something must be considered in order to understand its different parts
13) differentiate	m. matching or connected with something that you have just mentioned
14) manifestation	n. to recognize or show that two things are not the same
15) maintenance	o. the number of things or people that a container or space can hold

3. Fill in the blanks with the words from the box and change the form when necessary.

mental	pathological	nourishing	physiological	generalized
expounded	holism	manifestation	hermetic	disproved
capacity	maintain	therapeutic	collective	corresponding

1) He and his contemporaries — Plato and Aristotle — develop the concept of _____: the

mind and body are one, and medicine should treat both.

2) On its website, the Landing, a former motel near La Guardia Airport, describes itself as a temporary homeless shelter with a _____ for 169 families that is financed by the city's Department of Homeless Services.

3) She draws comparisons between the Internet and the natural world, making a case for the long-term _____ of self, community, and place, both online and off.

4) For older children and teens, you may see _____ changes, such as changes in sleep or appetite, reduced energy, or increased physical symptoms such as headaches or stomach-aches.

5) Her situation was further complicated and her vulnerability amplified (扩大) by _____ illness and substance abuse.

6) Thanks to a triple-threat of healthful ingredients, however, this soup gets its luxurious texture in a supremely _____ way with no cream at all.

7) The first _____ changes in the brain, the amyloid plaques (淀粉样斑块), appear up to 20 years before there is any cognitive impairment.

8) All my memories of my father include some _____ of his disability, even if none of us were quite willing to call it that yet.

9) In that now-viral video, Warren _____ on her economic theory of income distribution.

10) In this more complex view, patterns such as depression and _____ anxiety arise as tendencies in the human brain-body-environment system.

11) Isn't it true that it often happens that we think we've found something that appears unique in humans but those findings are later _____ ?

12) I always think of Emily's life as a very internal life in some ways, and a New England village inherently seems like a very _____ place.

13) "The development of vaccines and _____ is one important part of the research agenda. But it's only one part," he explained.

14) As scientists, engineers and health professionals, we see that this is our moment to bring our _____ knowledge to bear on this challenge and change the trajectory (轨道) of this response.

15) Whenever our kids wanted more autonomy (自主性), I always tried to combine that freedom with a _____ responsibility, a sense of ownership of it.

Task Three   Translation

1   Translate the following medical expressions into English

1) 藏象学说
2) 五脏六腑
3) 奇恒之腑
4) 鼻塞流涕
5) 传化水谷
6) 贮藏精气
7) 表里关系
8) 治疗效果
9) 临床实践
10) 藏而不泻

11）泻而不藏   12）满而不实
13）实而不满   14）精神情志活动
15）生理功能   16）病理变化
17）五脏属阴   18）六腑属阳
19）解剖概念   20）整体观念

2   Translate the following sentences into Chinese or English

1) The theory of visceral manifestation studies the physiological functions and pathological changes of viscera and their relations.

2) The common physiological function of the five *zang*-organs is to transform and store essence; while that of the six *fu*-organs is to receive, transport and transform water and food.

3) The related *fu*-organ can be purged for the treatment of the excess type of *zang*-organ disorders, and the related *zang*-organ can be nourished for the treatment of the deficiency type of *fu*-organ disorders.

4) The balance of the five *zang*-organs' physiological functions is the key to maintaining a relative constant internal environment of the human body.

5) The viscera in the theory of visceral manifestation is not only a simple anatomical concept, but also a concept that generalizes the physiology and pathology of a certain system.

6) 肝开窍于目,脾开窍于口。(open into)

7) 心与小肠相表里,心火过盛可随经络下移小肠。(internally and externally related to)

8) 阿是穴没有固定的部位和名称,也不归属于任何经脉。(pertain to)

9) 肺司呼吸,主通调水道,是机体抵御外邪的第一道防线。(be involved in)

10) 卫气营血辨证将外感温病划分为卫分证、气分证、营分证和血分证四个阶段。(be classified into)

3   Translate the following passage into English

　　人体是一个有机的整体。任一内脏均与形体诸窍具有特定的联系,因此内脏的生理功能、病理变化在外皆有一定的征象反映。通过考察相关的外在征象,即可推测内脏的功能状况。如通过观察面色、舌色、脉象等外在征象便可了解心之主血功能是否正常。

◥ Text B

The Liver: Properties and Functions

The liver stores the blood

1   Blood flow varies according to the time of day, the season of the year, a person's constitution, and the state of physical and mental quietude or agitation. Blood flows at a reduced rate when sleeping, and at an increased rate when physically working.

quietude /ˈkwaɪətjuːd/ *n*. 镇静

agitation /ˌædʒɪˈteɪʃən/ *n*. 躁动

Thirteen centuries ago, the influential Tang dynasty scholar Wang Bing described this function of the liver in the following manner: "The liver stores the blood, and the heart moves it. If a person moves about in a waking state, then the blood is distributed throughout all channels; if a person rests, the blood returns to the liver."

2   Emotions such as anger, embarrassment, or unexpected joy can also increase blood flow, causing the ears and face to turn red. In situations when less blood is needed, it is "stored in the liver," which thus assumes a warehouse-like function. The actual storage of blood is done in the **penetrating** vessel, one of the eight **extraordinary** vessels that extends from the lower *dantian* to the head; this vessel is often considered to be part of the liver network. The liver is best compared to a managing clerk, who moves goods in and out of the **warehouse** as they are needed.

penetrate /'penətreɪt/ *v.* 刺入

extraordinary /ɪk'strɔː(r)dənərɪ/ *adj.* 非凡的

warehouse /'weə(r)haʊs/ *n.* 仓库

The liver is in charge of coursing and draining

3   Just as important is the liver's function of maintaining a smooth and uninterrupted flow of **virtually** all body substances (including *qi*, blood, *jing*, and liquids and humors). The term *shu* (sometimes translated as coursing or smoothing) is used to refer to the action of maintaining a mode of operation in the body that is not **stagnating**, not overly agitated, and continuously flowing. The term *xie* (sometimes translated as draining) is used to refer to the liver's action of purging stagnation in the spleen/stomach. Proper coursing and draining, or lack **thereof**, is mostly reflected in the relation of emotions to *qi* and blood circulation and to the influence of the liver on **digestive** system functions:

virtually /'vɜː(r)tʃuəlɪ/ *adv.* 几乎

stagnate /stæg'neɪt/ *v.* 淤塞

thereof /ˌðeər'ɒv/ *adv.* 它的

digestive /daɪ'dʒestɪv/ *adj.* 消化的

4   Emotional aspect: the ancient Chinese observed that human emotions are largely governed by the heart network. However, they also concluded that mental well-being or various shades of depression have an association with the coursing and draining function of the liver. Only if the liver carries this task out properly can the body's *qi* and blood flow unobstructedly, and thus **facilitate** a feeling of ease, harmony, and peace. If for some reason the liver fails to maintain this state, depression (of liver *qi*) or pathological rising (of liver *yang*) may result. As the Qing Dynasty classic, *Xue Zheng Lun* (*A Treatise on Blood Disorders*), states: "The liver is classified as wood; wood *qi* is characterized by its

facilitate /fə'sɪlɪteɪt/ *v.* 促进

determination to go straight to where it wants to go to; if it is not blocked or suppressed, the movement in the vessels will be smooth."

5　Digestive aspect: since this moving function of the liver regulates the *qi* flow in the entire body, it influences the dynamics of the other organ networks, particularly the neighboring digestive systems. It assists the upward and downward flows of the spleen/ stomach system (the stomach is to move the food mass downward, the spleen is to move the extracted *qi* upward), passes **bile** into the **intestines**, helps to transport food essence, and aids the unobstructed movement and metabolism of water. The *Xue Zheng Lun* says "Coursing and draining is an integral part of the nature of liver. Once food *qi* enters the stomach, it is entirely up to the liver wood to course and drain it. Only if this process is intact will grain and water transform properly."

bile /baɪl/ *n*. 胆汁

intestine /ɪnˈtestɪn/ *n*. 肠

The liver is in charge of the tendons and manifests in the nails

6　The **tendons** connect the muscles to the bones. In accordance with the characteristics of the liver, they facilitate smooth and continuous movement. Because of this basic concept, some scholars have recently included the nerves (which do not have a separate designation in classical Chinese theory) under the category "tendons" (*jin*). The proper functioning of the tendons relies entirely on their nourishment by liver blood.

tendon /ˈtendən/ *n*. 筋

7　The nails are considered the **surplus** of the tendons. As such, they are an exterior manifestation of the general quality of the tendons, and thus, liver blood within. Dry and **brittle** or extremely pale nail beds always indicate a poor quality of liver blood, while pink nail beds and firm nails indicate a healthy state of liver blood.

surplus /ˈsɜː(r)pləs/ *n*. 剩余

brittle /ˈbrɪtl/ *adj*. 脆的

8　Hair is also associated with the liver blood: it is called the "surplus of the blood" (*xue yu*). The rich liver blood of females is expressed in lush, long, and fast-growing hair on the head; males have more facial and body hair, which is governed by the *qi* organ, lung. Dry and brittle hair can be an indication of liver blood deficiency, while hair that suddenly falls out (**alopecia**) is usually because of both deficiency of blood and impeded flow of liver blood to the head, usually due to sudden emotional trauma.

alopecia /ˌæləˈpiːʃə/ *n*. 脱发

The liver has its opening in the eyes

9   The eyes are nourished by the essence of all five organ networks, and thus differentiated into five organ specific zones which may reveal important diagnostic information. The eyes as a whole, however, represent the opening of the liver, and are thus considered to be more closely linked to the liver than to any of the other organ networks. "Liver *qi* communicates with the eyes," states the *Neijing*, "and if the liver functions harmoniously, the eyes can differentiate the five essential colors." If the liver receives blood, we can see. The liver channel branches out to the eyes. Both liver *qi* and liver blood flood the eyes to maintain proper eyesight. A person's eyesight may therefore also serve as an indicator for liver function.

The liver is in charge of planning and strategy, and the gallbladder is in charge of decision making

10   Just as trees (wood) tend to **unrelentingly** pursue their upward quest for the light, the liver represents the innate will of the body/mind to spread outward. Just like *qi* and blood have to spread within the body to ensure physical survival, human *shen* needs to spread freely through the social environment to guarantee an uninhibited passage through life. Individuals with strong liver *qi* and sufficient blood are usually excellent strategic planners and decision makers: they know how to spread themselves into the world. Due to these qualities, they often become outstanding business managers. If, however, this tough and determined spreading nature of the liver is not in a state of harmonious balance with the softer side of liver wood, ease, smoothness, and flexibility, then the wood-endangering state of **rigidity** arises. (1,096 words)

(adapted from http://www.itmonline.org/5organs/liver.htm)

unrelentingly /ˌʌnrɪˈlentɪŋlɪ/ *adv*. 不屈不挠地

rigidity /rɪˈdʒɪdətɪ/ *n*. 强直

Notes:

1. "The liver stores the blood, and the heart moves it. If a person moves about in a waking state, then the blood is distributed throughout all channels; if a person rests, the blood returns to the liver." "肝藏血,心行之,人动则血运于诸经,人静则血归于肝脏。"

2. penetrating vessel: 冲脉。

3. coursing or smoothing: 疏。

4. depression (of liver *qi*): 肝气郁结。

5. pathological rising (of liver *yang*)：肝阳上亢。

6. "The liver is classified as wood; wood *qi* is characterized by its determination to go straight to where it wants to go to; if it is not blocked or suppressed, the movement in the vessels will be smooth." "肝属木,木气冲和条达,不致遏郁,则血脉得畅。"

7. "Coursing and draining is an integral part of liver the nature of. Once food *qi* enters the stomach, it is entirely up to the liver wood to course and drain it. Only if this process is intact will grain and water transform properly." "木之性主于疏泄,食气入胃,全赖肝木之气以疏泄之,而水谷乃化。"

8. dry and brittle 干脆易折

9. surplus of the blood 血余

10. "Liver *qi* communicates with the eyes, and if the liver functions harmoniously, the eyes can differentiate the five essential colors." "肝气通于目,肝和则目能辨五色矣。"

11. The liver is in charge of coursing and draining. 肝主疏泄。

12. The liver is in charge of the tendons and manifests in the nails. 肝主筋,其华在爪。

13. The liver has its opening in the eyes. 肝开窍于目。

14. The liver is in charge of planning and strategy, and the gallbladder is in charge of decision making. 肝主谋略,胆主决断。

Task One   Reading Comprehension

1. According to the text, which is NOT a factor affecting the blood flow?

    A. The time of day.

    B. A person's inclination.

    C. The season of the year.

    D. A person's emotions.

2. The nails are considered an exterior manifestation of the general quality of the _____ .

    A. blood   B. essence   C. tendons   D. *qi*

3. According to the theory of visceral manifestation, all sayings are correct about the characteristics of liver EXCEPT _____ .

    A. opening in the eyes   B. in charge of decision making

    C. in charge of the tendons   D. in charge of smoothing

4. The actual storage of blood is done in the _____ .

    A. conception vessel   B. governor vessel

    C. belt vessel   D. penetrating vessel

5. Why have the nerves recently been included under the category "tendons" (*jin*)?

    A. Because the tendons promote smooth and continuous movement.

    B. Because the tendons connect the bones to the muscles.

    C. Because the tendons' characteristics are inconsistent with that of the liver.

    D. Because the tendons' functions rely on their nourishment by liver *qi*.

Task Two   Vocabulary

1. Directions: Complete the following phrases respectively according to its corresponding meaning or equivalent in Chinese within the brackets.

1) _____(静) or _____(躁)

2) liver blood _____(不足)

3) *qi* and blood _____(循环)

4) _____(津) and _____(液)

5) a _____(仓库样的) function

6) _____(消化系统)

7) eight _____(八脉)

8) _____vessel (冲脉)

9) _____(郁结) of liver *qi*

10) _____(上亢) of liver *yang*

11) _____(动态) of the liver networks

12) transport _____(食物精微)

13) dry and _____(易折的) nails

14) _____(茂密的) and fast growing hair

15) _____(脱发症)

16) sudden emotional _____(创伤)

17) _____(诊断的) information

18) maintain proper _____(视力)

19) _____(策略规划者)

20) _____(决策者)

2. Fill in the blanks with the words from the box and change the form when necessary.

substance	drain	uninterrupted	stagnate	innate
unobstructed	trauma	smooth	metabolism	impeded
extracted	relent	indicate	intact	circulate

1) Doctors should stop relying on weight alone as a(n) _____ of health and slavishly (亦步亦趋地) prescribing weight loss to treat health ailments.

2) She says he's been dealing with depression along with _____ brain jury.

3) "Usually the signs of infection are pretty easy to identify. It's like fire-engine red around your toe, if it's warm, if it's _____ pus(脓), if it's painful to touch — those are all signs of infections."

4) In 2018, the FDA issued a warning about hair _____ products containing formaldehyde(甲醛), but was powerless to recall or ban them.

5) The study, "Uninterrupted Infant Sleep, Development, and Maternal Mood," defined a full night of sleep as between 6 and 8 hours without _____.

6) The researchers say that while some of the _____ may also be found in animal or plant matter, no such remains were reported during excavations(挖掘).

7) When the heart stops and blood stops _____, the brain quickly becomes starved of oxygen, suffering irreparable damage within about five minutes.

8) She developed two small-bowel _____, and each surgery was followed by significant cognitive decline and delirium(精神错乱).

9) At the same time, fever caused by the virus increases the body's _____ and the heart's output of blood.

10) Although tooth enamel(牙釉质) offers the best source of acidic proteins, researchers are also

_____ them from bones and hair.

11) This is an accumulation and _____ of the blood in one of the organs, usually in the brain, though occasionally in the lungs.

12) Salles told Reuters on Thursday that the majority of the Amazon remains _____ , showing that Brazil is doing an "excellent job" to preserve the environment.

13) Researchers tend to view inflammation as a(n) _____ to regenerative healing.

14) Under increasing pressure, the FDA _____ and removed many of the bureaucratic obstacles.

15) The _____ immune system on which they rely was long thought to provide a fast but non-specific response to pathogens, and considered unable to use experience of previous attacks to improve protection in the future.

Task Three   Writing

Please rewrite the text in a form of abstract (about 150 words).

Terminology

本书配套数字教学资源

Basic Terminology of Visceral Manifestation

Terminology	WHO	WFCMS
脏腑	viscera and bowls	*zang-fu* organs
奇恒之腑	extraordinary organ	extraordinary *fu*-organ
三焦	triple energizers	triple energizer; CO (17); triple energizer (sanjiao)
胞	placenta	uterus; placenta; eyelid; urinary bladder
脑户	back of the head	back of head; GV 17 (Naohu)
神明	bright spirit	mental activity; bright spirit
血脉	blood vessel	blood and vessels
产门,阴户,阴门	无	vaginal orifice
天癸	heavenly tenth	reproduction-stimulating essence
治节	management and regulation	management and regulation
元神之府	house of the original spirit	house of original spirit
水之上源	upper source of water	upper source of water
心肾相交	heart-kidney interaction	heart-kidney interaction
肝肾同源	homogeny of liver and kidney	liver and kidney from same source
泌别清浊	separation of the clear and turbid	separating lucid and turbid
膀胱气化	bladder *qi* transformation	bladder *qi* transformation

The moving influences between the kidneys constitute
a person's root and foundation.

气者，人之根本也①。

Unit 4　　*Qi*，　Blood，　Body fluids and Essence

Warming-up

Before you listen（Watch）

In this section you will hear a short passage about "What is *Qi*". The following words and phrases may be of help.

bioelectric /ˌbaɪəʊɪlek'trɪk/	*a*.	生物电的
prescientific /ˌprɪsaɪən'tɪfɪk/	*a*.	近代科学出现以前的,科学发展以前的
predate /ˌpriː'deɪt/	*v*.	在日期上早于(先于)
Newtonian /njuː'təʊnɪən/	*a*.	牛顿(学说)的
penetrate /'penətreɪt/	*v*.	渗透,穿透,洞察
galaxy /'ɡæləksɪ/	*n*.	星系,银河系
pathogen /'pæθədʒən/	*n*.	病原体,病菌
bacteria /bæk'tɪərɪə/	*n*.	细菌
hearty /'hɑːtɪ/	*a*.	丰盛的,健壮的
allergy /'ælədʒɪ/	*n*.	过敏症;厌恶
irritable /'ɪrɪtəbl/	*a*.	过敏的;急躁的,易怒的
mindfulness /'maɪndflnəs/	*n*.	正念;留心,警觉
meditation /ˌmedɪ'teɪʃn/	*n*.	冥想,沉思,静坐

---

① 《难经·八难》,Paul U. Unschuld 译。

While you listen (Watch)

Listen to the passage carefully and fill in each of the blanks marked from 1) to 10) according to what you have heard.

There are several different types of *qi* in the body, and all of them can be either 1) _____ , excess or deficient in nature.

There are five major functions of *qi*. The first one is to protect the body. *Qi* will protect the body from 2) _____ pathogens, such as heat, cold, 3) _____ , dryness, and also bacteria, viruses, and other types of pathogens. *Qi* also has a warming function. It warms and cools the body as needed. It also has a holding function, where it holds the organs in place, keeps blood in the blood vessels, and governs all the 4) _____ . It also has a transformation function where it converts food and air into *qi* and blood. It's also responsible for 5) _____ , and it governs all the movement of *qi* and blood through the meridians and prevents stagnation and promotes growth.

If you have good *qi*, you're going to feel energetic. You'll have good endurance, strong but relaxed muscles, a balanced immune system, fast healing, a hearty digestion, a clear mind, and good 6) _____ . And you'll sleep well.

If your *qi* is deficient, you'll feel low energy. You'll have a weak or overactive immune system. You'll have allergies and 7) _____ , depression, slow healing, poor digestion, poor appetite, weight gain, poor concentration and poor memory.

If you have excess *qi*, you'll feel irritable, stressed. You have tight muscles and headaches, poor sleep, pain — that's worse with pressure, tight jaw and shallow 8) _____ .

Here are four tips for healthy *qi*. The first one is to move your body. If you are deficient, move only about 20 minutes a day. This can be walking, light exercise, dancing, swimming. And if you are excess in nature, you need higher 9) _____ and more exercise. The second tip is to feed your body correctly depending on whether you are excess or deficient. We may go into this in a future video. The third tip is to practice Qi Gong, Tai Chi, Yoga and mindfulness 10) _____ . All of these help advance the *qi* very quickly and easily. And the last tip, which is possibly the most important, is to do something that you really enjoy every single day for about 15 minutes.

After you listen(Watch)

Please discuss with your partner the following questions and give your presentation to the class.

1) How does the ancient Chinese philosophy see *qi*?
2) What's your understanding of *qi* dynamic/ movement (*qi* ji) in TCM?
3) What's the so-called primordial *qi* (yuan *qi*) in TCM?
4) How does *qi* and blood affect each other according to TCM?

Reading

 Text A

BEFORE CLASS

1. Quest for Definition

Directions：Explore online the definitions of the following terms from Text A and prepare a unique _one-minute_ oral presentation for your class.

1) innate _qi_ and acquired _qi_

2) _qi_ movement/dynamic

3) categories of _qi_

4) physiological functions of _qi_

5) blood in TCM

6) body fluids in TCM

2. Text-based Activities

Directions：Read carefully the part of Text A that corresponds to your task，and then prepare a unique _one-minute_ oral presentation for your class.

PERFORMANCE IN CLASS

Your Task

1) What is pectoral _qi_ in TCM?

2) What is nutrient _qi_ in TCM?

3) What's the defending function of _qi_?

4) How is _qi_ generated according to TCM?

5) What are physiological functions of body fluids according to TCM?

_Qi_, Blood and Body Fluids [①]

1　_Qi_, blood and body fluids are the basic substances that **constitute** the human body and maintain life activities. Their production and metabolism depend upon the functional activities of the viscera, meridians, organs and tissues.

---

① Body Fluids：“津液”，也常译作 humor，或 body fluid，由于津液包括人体各种器官和组织的分泌物，应用复数形式，故本文采用 body fluids。

I. *Qi*

2　*Qi* in TCM is the most essential substance to constitute the human body and sustain its life activity. *Qi* in the body is derived from innate *qi* (xian tian zhi *qi*)① that is transformed from the kidney essence inherited from the parents, and acquired *qi* (hou tian zhi *qi*)② from both food nutrients that are transformed by the spleen and stomach and fresh air that is inhaled by the lung. The production of *qi* depends on the **synthetic** actions of the viscera, especially the kidney, spleen, stomach and lung. *Qi* is powerful in activity and flows constantly in the body to maintain the physiological functions of the body. Such a constant motion of *qi* is called *qi* movement. The styles of *qi* movement③ are theoretically summarized as ascending, descending, exiting and entering. The viscera and meridians are the places where the activities of *qi* take place. According to the composition, distribution and functions, *qi* is mainly divided into four categories, namely **primordial** *qi* (yuan *qi*)④, **pectoral** *qi* (zong *qi*)⑤, nutrient *qi* (ying *qi*)⑥ and defensive *qi* (wei *qi*)⑦.

3　There are mainly five physiological functions of *qi*. The first function is promoting. *Qi* is a vigorous and refined substance with powerful activity. It promotes and stimulates the growth and development of the human body, physiological activities of the viscera and meridians, the production and circulation of blood as well as the production, distribution and **excretion** of body fluids. The second physiological function of *qi* is warming. *Qi* is the source of energy of the body. This is prerequisite to the maintenance of normal body temperature, normal physiological activities of the viscera and normal circulation of blood and body fluids. The third function of *qi* is defending. The defending system of the body is complicated, however, *qi* plays a very important role in it. Under the healthy condition, defensive *qi* in the body surface will consolidate the **striae and interstices** ⑧ to prevent invasion of exogenous pathogenic factors. Under abnormal conditions, healthy *qi* (zheng *qi*)⑨ can fight against pathogenic *qi* (xie *qi*)⑩, driving it away to cure disease. The fourth physiological function of *qi* is consolidating. *Qi* can prevent blood from **extravasation** and regulate the secretion and excretion of sweat, urine, saliva, **gastric** juices, intestinal fluids and sperm in order to avoid unnecessary loss. The fifth and final function of *qi* is transforming. This action refers to the metabolism and mutual transformation of essence, *qi*, blood and body fluids. For instance, the production of *qi*, blood and body fluids depend on the transformation of food

---

①　innate *qi* (xian tian zhi *qi*)：先天之气。
②　acquired *qi* (hou tian zhi *qi*)：后天之气。
③　*qi* movement,亦常作 *qi* dynamic、*qi* activity,气机。
④　primordial *qi* (yuan *qi*)：元气,在中医还常作原气、真气。
⑤　pectoral *qi* (zong *qi*)：宗气,英语中还常译作 ancestral *qi*。
⑥　nutrient *qi* (ying *qi*)：营气,英语中还常译作 nutritive *qi*。
⑦　defensive *qi* (wei *qi*)：卫气,英语中还常译作 defense *qi*。
⑧　striae and interstices：腠理。腠,指肌肉的纹理,又称肌腠,即肌纤维间的空隙;理,指皮肤的纹理,即皮肤之间的缝隙。故腠理一般指肌肉和皮肤的纹理。
⑨　healthy *qi* (zheng *qi*)：正气,英语中还常译作 vital *qi* 等。
⑩　pathogenic *qi* (xie *qi*)：邪气,英语中还常译作 pathogenic factors、evil *qi* 等。

into nutrients; body fluids are converted into sweat and urine by means of metabolism; and after digestion and absorption, the residues of food turn into feces. All these processes are the concrete **manifestations** of the transforming action of *qi*.

II. Blood

4　Blood is a red liquid substance rich in nutrients and circulating in the vessels. It is one of the indispensable materials to form the human body and maintain its vital activities. Blood is primarily composed of nutrient *qi* and body fluids which come mainly from food nutrients transformed by the spleen and stomach. This is why the spleen and stomach are considered as the source of *qi* and blood and also play an important role in the production of blood. Since the nutrient *qi* and body fluids come from the nutrients of the foodstuff, so the quality of food and the functions of the spleen and stomach directly influence the production of blood. In addition, the essence stored in the kidney is also an essential substance to promote blood production. That is why it is said that "the essence and blood share the same origin①".

5　The main physiological function of the blood is to nourish and moisten the whole body. The blood circulates inside the vessels throughout the body, internally to the viscera and externally to the skin, muscles, tendons and bones. It flows continuously and ceaselessly to nourish and moisten all the organs and tissues to maintain their normal physiological functions. The nourishing and moistening functions of the blood are signified by such external manifestations as rosy **complexion**, well-developed and strong muscles, lustrous skin and hair as well as nimble and flexible sensation and movement. Blood is also the material basis for the mental activities. Therefore, it is said in *Ling Shu* (*Miraculous Pivot*) that "the harmony of blood and smoothness of the vessels are key to the normal state of the spirit②."

III. Body Fluids

6　Body fluids are a collective term for all kinds of normal liquids in the body, including secretions from various organs and tissues, such as gastric juice, **intestinal** fluids, nasal discharge, tears, sweat and urine, etc. Body fluids are derived from the food that is transported and transformed by the spleen and stomach. According to the difference in quality, function and distribution, it is subdivided into two: jin (thin fluid)③ and ye (thick fluid)④. Generally speaking, thin fluid mainly spreads in the skin, muscles and orifices, and penetrates into the vessels as a component of blood.

---

①　the essence and blood share the same origin：精血同源。

②　the harmony of blood and smoothness of the vessels are key to the normal state of the spirit："血脉和利,精神乃居",语出《灵枢·平人绝谷》；*Ling Shu*（*Miraculous Pivot*），《灵枢》，英语中还常译作 *Spiritual Pivot*。

③　jin (thin fluid)：津。中医一般将质地较清稀,流动性较大,布散于体表皮肤、肌肉和孔窍,并能渗入血脉之内,起滋润作用的体液称为津。

④　ye (thick fluid)：液。中医一般将质地较浓稠,流动性较小,灌注于骨节、脏腑、脑、髓等,起濡养作用的体液称为液。

Thick fluid supports in the skeleton, joints, viscera, and brain. There is no difference in nature of these fluids and liquids, so they are often collectively termed as "body fluids".

7　The production, distribution and excretion of body fluids are a complicated physiological process involving multiple viscera. The physiological functions of body fluids include moistening and nourishing the body, transforming and enriching blood, regulating *yin* and *yang*, **neutralizing toxin and excreting waste**. (926 words)

New Words and Expressions

constitute /ˈkɒnstɪtjuːt/ *vt*. to be the parts that together form something 组成,构成

synthetic /sɪnˈθetɪk/ *adj*. involving or of the nature of synthesis (combining separate elements to form a coherent whole) 综合的

primordial /praɪˈmɔːdɪəl/ *adj*. existing at the beginning of time or the beginning of the Earth 原始的,原生的,根本的

pectoral /ˈpektərəl/ *adj*. relating to or connected with the chest or breast 胸的

excretion /ɪkˈskriːʃn/ *n*. the act of passing solid or liquid waste matter from the body 排泄,排泄物; 分泌,分泌物

striae /ˈstraɪiː/ *n*. a striped pattern on something, especially on a muscle 条纹

interstice /ɪnˈtɜːstɪs/ *n*. a small space or crack in something or between things 空隙

extravasation /ɛkˌstrævəˈseʃən/ *n*. an extravasated liquid (blood or lymph or urine); the product of extravasation 溢出,溢出物

gastric /ˈɡæstrɪk/ *adj*. relating to or involving the stomach 胃的,胃部的

manifestation /ˌmænɪfeˈsteɪʃn/ *n*. the act of appearing as a sign that something exists or is happening 表现,显示

complexion /kəmˈplekʃn/ *n*. the natural colour and condition of the skin on a person's face 肤色,面色

intestinal /ɪnˈtestɪnl/ *adj*. of or relating to or inside the intestines 肠的

neutralize /ˈnjuːtrəlaɪz/ *vt*. to make ineffective by counterbalancing the effect of 抵销,使……中和,使……无效

FOLLOW-UP ACTIVITIES

Task one　Comprehension Check

1. Questions for Discussion

1) How meridians and *qi* act upon each other according to TCM?

2) Why does our body temperature remain comparatively stable?

3) Can you briefly explain how *qi* transforms according to TCM?

4) Why do we divide body fluids into jin (thin fluid) and ye (thick fluid) clinically?

2. Chart Completion

INTRODUCTION: (para. 1)

The production and metabolism of *qi* , blood and body fluids depend upon the 1) _____ _____ of the viscera, meridians, organs and tissues.

CATEGORIES AND PHYSIOLOGICAL FUNCTIONS OF QI: (para. 2 – 3)

Four categories of *qi* in TCM: primordial *qi* (yuan *qi*), pectoral *qi* (zong *qi*), 2) _____ _____ and defensive *qi* (wei *qi*).

Five physiological functions of *qi* in TCM:

- Qi 3) _____ the growth and development of the human body. The physiological activities of the Zang-Fu organs and meridians, the production and circulation of blood as well as 4) _____ of body fluids all depend on *qi* .

- 5) _____ is the prerequisite to the maintenance of our normal body temperature, that's why we do not feel so cold even in winter days.

- Under normal conditions, our human body surface will consolidate the striae and interstices to prevent invasion of the exogenous pathogenic factors; under abnormal conditions, healthy *qi* (zheng *qi*) can drive away pathogenic *qi* (xie *qi*) to restore our health all because of 6) _____ .

- The consolidating function of *qi* prevents blood from spilling out and helps to regulate the 7) _____ of sweat, urine, saliva, gastric juice, intestinal juice, sperm, etc.

- Due to the transforming function of *qi* , the metabolism and mutual transformation of 8) _____ occur.

GENERATION AND PHYSIOLOGICAL FUNCTIONS OF BLOOD: (para. 4 – 5)

Generation of blood in TCM:

Mainly composed of 9) _____ which comes mainly from food nutrients which are transformed by the 10) _____ , blood forms the human body and maintains its life activities as one of the indispensable materials.

Physiological functions of blood in TCM:

Blood flows continuously and ceaselessly to 11) _____ all the organs and tissues to maintain their normal physiological functions, which in return gives us ruddy complexion, well-developed and strong muscles, lustrous skin and hair, nimble and flexible sensation and movement.

GENERATION AND PHYSIOLOGICAL FUNCTIONS OF BODY FLUIDS: (para. 6 – 7)

Generation of body fluids in TCM:

As different kinds of normal liquids, body fluids are derived from 12) _____ _____ mainly transported and transformed by the spleen and stomach, which is quite similar to the production of blood in the human body.

Physiological functions of body fluids in TCM:

The physiological functions of body fluids are multifold, including moistening and nourishing the body, 13) _____ blood, regulating *yin* and *yang*, neutralizing toxin and excreting waste. Because body fluids and blood are both derived from the food we have and they will be transformed into each other when necessary, that's why we often say 14) _____ .

Task Two   Vocabulary

1. **Directions: Complete the following phrases respectively according to its corresponding meaning or equivalent in Chinese within the brackets.**

1) _____ （元气）

2) food _____（精微）

3) _____（生成）of blood

4) _____ （输布）of body fluids

5) consolidate _____ （腠理）

6) prevent invasion of _____（外邪）

7) _____（正气）fighting against pathogenic *qi*

8) _____（卫气）

9) _____（消化）and absorption

10) digestion and_____ （吸收）

11) the _____ （糟粕）of food

12) an _____ （必要的）substance

13) the _____ （濡润）functions

14) the _____（分泌排泄）of sweat

15) the ruddy _____（脸色）

16) _____（有光泽的）skin and hair

17) the material _____（基础）

18) the _____ （和利）of blood and the vessels

19) _____ （津）

20) _____ （液）

2. **Match the following words with their proper meanings.**

Column I	Column II
1) metabolism	a. (of a quality, feeling, etc.) that you have when you are born
2) innate	b. in a theoretical manner
3) inhale	c. internal organs collectively (especially those in the abdominal cavity)
4) invasion	d. the chemical processes by which food is changed into energy in your body
5) theoretically	e. draw deep into the lungs in by breathing

continued

Column I	Column II
6) viscera	f. any entry into an area not previously occupied
7) meridian	g. something that must exist or happen before sth. else can happen or be done
8) composition	h. strengthen; make sth. stronger or more solid
9) prerequisite	i. (of a disease or symptom) having a cause that is outside the body
10) consolidate	j. any of several bodily processes by which substances go out of the body
11) exogenous	k. waste matter (as urine or sweat but especially feces) discharged from the body
12) discharge	l. any substance that is used as food
13) nimble	m. moving quickly and lightly
14) secreta	n. the way in which something is made up of different parts, things, or members
15) foodstuff	o. an imaginary great circle on the surface of the earth passing through the north and south poles at right angles to the equator; any of the pathways along which the body's vital energy flows according to the theory behind acupuncture

3. Fill in the blanks with the words from the box and change the form when necessary.

synthetic	inhale	foodstuff	viscera	meridian
composition	primordial	exogenous	gastric	neutralize
pathogenic	excretion	intestinal	nimble	theoretically

1) The method of the practical philosopher consists, therefore, of two processes: analytical and _____.

2) The researchers asked what would happen if calories in the diet were kept constant but the carbohydrate _____ of a diet varied from high to very low.

3) Further testing is under way to determine the strain and whether the virus is highly _____.

4) She _____ deeply and threw her head back to blow the smoke towards the ceiling.

5) Scientists on Monday announced the discovery in the Australian outback of fossils of this creature that represents one of the most important _____ animals ever found.

6) The disease spreads through animal-to-animal contact and indirectly through food and soil contaminated with bodily _____.

7) Now, industrialized countries are almost self-sufficient in basic _____ due to the use of fertilizers, mechanization and larger farm units.

8) Swine flu is just the latest in a series of "_____ events" (risks originating outside the financial system) to test the markets.

9) She also suffered from hair loss and _____ parasites.

10) After his death, all the abdominal _____ were found in a state of ulceration (溃疡).

11) Patients with conditions such as _____ ulcers may be prescribed medicine to reduce the acidity in the stomach to relieve unpleasant symptoms.

12) Physical fitness may be critical for maintaining a relatively youthful and _____ brain as we age, according to a new study of brain activation patterns in older people.

13) _____ disease and collateral disease are two different categories of pathological changes.

14) Once there, given enough time, these disinfectants will damage the virus, _____ it.

15) The goal of these operations was straightforward: to remove as many cancer cells as possible, which would _____ prolong the survival of patients and possibly even cure them.

Task Three   Translation

1. Translate the following medical expressions into English

1) 基本物质   2) 功能活动

3) 气机   4) 后天之气

5) 营气   6) 胃气

7) 脏腑经络   8) 血液运行

9) 津液排泄   10) 外感病邪

11) 具体表现   12) 生理功能

13) 精血同源   14) 血脉和利

15) 面色红润   16) 肌肉强健

2. Translate the following sentences into Chinese or English

1) The production of *qi* depends on the synthetic actions of the viscera, especially the kidney, spleen, stomach and lung.

2) According to the composition, distribution and functions, *qi* is mainly divided into four categories, namely primordial *qi* (yuan *qi*), pectoral *qi* (zong *qi*), nutrient *qi* (ying *qi*) and defensive *qi* (wei *qi*).

3) This is prerequisite to the maintenance of normal body temperature, normal physiological activities of the viscera and normal circulation of blood and body fluids.

4) Since the nutrient *qi* and body fluids come from the nutrients of the foodstuff, the quality of food and the functions of the spleen and stomach directly influence the production of blood.

5) Body fluids are a collective term for all kinds of normal liquids in the body, including secreta from various organs and tissues, such as gastric juice, intestinal juice, nasal discharge, tears, sweat and urine, etc.

6) 不要因为想要忘掉痛苦的回忆或者安慰自己而养成暴饮暴食的恶习。(drive away)

7) 医学专家说,一般情况下,快递包裹在运输过程中被新型冠状病毒污染的可能性不大。(under normal conditions)

8) 在意大利,医院和卫生人员超负荷工作,政府已经开始将酒店改造成方舱医院来收治轻症新型冠状病毒感染的肺炎患者。(convert ... into)

9) 如果是在常规临床护理、一般的工作生活条件下,采取佩戴口罩的飞沫传播防护措施,是足以保护普通公众不被感染的。(prevent ... from)

10) 外感病发病与否除时令外邪的致病因素外,还与人体上呼吸道微生态平衡有关。(exogenous

pathogenic factors)

3. Translate the following passage into English

中国古代朴素的"元气论"认为元气是构成宇宙万物的最本质、最原始的要素,其源头可追溯到老子的"道"。按照元气论,万物的产生、发展、变化和灭亡都是元气循"道"(即自然规律)而运动的结果。气为万物之精微,完全连续而无处不在。

◥ Text B

Relationships among *Qi*, Blood and Body Fluids

1 *Qi*, blood and body fluids are all the essential substances to form the body and maintain vital activities. They are all acquired from food nutrients that are transformed and absorbed by the spleen and stomach. Although different in nature and function, they are closely related to each other and promote each other in physiology, and also mutually affect and transmit during **pathology**. Therefore, it is very important to understand the relationships among *qi*, blood and body fluids.

pathology /pəˈθɒlədʒɪ/ *n.* 病理学

I. Relationships Between *Qi* and Blood

2 *Qi* pertains to *yang* while blood to *yin*. The relationships between *qi* and blood are usually generalized as "*qi* is the commander of blood and blood is the mother of *qi*".

3 *Qi* **generates** blood. This means that *qi* participates in and promotes blood production in various aspects. In terms of the composition, the **nutritive** *qi* (ying *qi*) can generate blood, and becomes a component of blood. In terms of the process of blood production, *qi* transformation of the viscera is the driving force for blood production. Food nutrients and kidney essence can both be transformed into blood. However, the entire process of blood production depends on *qi* transformation of the spleen, stomach, heart, lung and kidney. Sufficient nutritive *qi* and visceral *qi* (zang fu zhi *qi*) thereby generate sufficient blood to meet the body's needs, while **deficient** nutritive *qi* and visceral *qi* will lead to blood deficiency.

generate /ˈdʒenəreɪt/ *vt.* 使形成,生成
nutritive /ˈnjuːtrɪtɪv/ *a.* 有营养的,滋养的

deficient /dɪˈfɪʃnt/ *a.* 不足的,短缺的

4 *Qi* propels blood. Blood depends on the propelling action of *qi* to circulate and distribute to the whole body. Normal flow of *qi* ensures normal circulation of blood while **stagnation** of *qi* leads to

stagnation /stæɡˈneɪʃn/ *n.* 停滞

stasis of blood. In normal blood circulation, the heart *qi* is the driving force for blood circulation; the lung *qi* assists the heart to propel blood to circulate inside the vessels; and the liver *qi* keeps the blood circulation smooth. If *qi* fails to propel or stagnates, it will lead to **retarded** blood circulation or blood stasis.

5   *Qi* commands blood to circulate inside vessels to avoid bleeding. This is mainly related to the action of spleen *qi*. If spleen *qi* becomes deficient and fails to command blood, it can lead to various hemorrhages, such as hematuria, hematochezia and metrorrhagia.

6   Blood generates *qi*. This means that blood can nourish the *qi* of the body. Physiological functions of viscera depend on promoting, warming and transforming actions of visceral *qi*. Sufficient blood ensures sufficient *qi* while insufficient blood leads to *qi* deficiency.

7   Blood carries *qi*. This means that blood is a carrier of *qi*. Since *qi* pertains to *yang* and is very vigorous and active, it tends to **disperse**. So it must depend on blood as its carrier.

II. Relationships Between Qi and Body Fluids

8   *Qi* pertains to *yang* while body fluid to *yin*. The relationships between *qi* and body fluids are quite similar to the relationships between *qi* and blood.

9   *Qi* generates body fluids. This means that transformation of *qi* can promote generation of body fluids. Body fluids come from the water and food transformed by the spleen and stomach. Therefore the spleen and stomach play an important role in the production of body fluids. Sufficient *qi* of the spleen and stomach with **prosperous** *qi* transformation can generate sufficient body fluids, while deficient *qi* of the spleen and stomach with **hypoactive** *qi* transformation will lead to dysfunction in the generation of body fluids in generation, resulting in deficiency of body fluids.

10   *Qi* promotes the flow of body fluids. Body fluids are generated by the spleen and stomach, and are distributed to the whole body by visceral *qi*. In the process of metabolizing the of body fluids, the waste and surplus water are transformed into sweat and urine by *qi* transformation. Therefore, either *qi* deficiency or *qi* stagnation can cause disorder of body fluids in distribution, resulting in pathological products such as fluid

retarded /rɪ'tɑːdɪd/ *a*. 滞后的,弱智的

disperse /dɪ'spɜːs/ *vt*. 分散, 使散开

prosperous /'prɒspərəs/ *a*. 繁荣的,兴旺的

hypoactive /haɪpə(ʊ)'æktɪv/ *a*. 活动(力)减退的

retention, **phlegm** and dampness.

11　*Qi* controls body fluids. This is related to the regulating activities of opening and closing. Opening means to excrete the waste and surplus, part of body fluids out of the body, and closing means to keep the needed fluids in the body. For example, lung *qi* and defensive *qi* （wei *qi*) can regulate sweat, spleen *qi* and kidney *qi* can regulate saliva, and kidney *qi* and **bladder** *qi* can regulate urine.

12　Body fluids carry *qi*. Body fluids are also a carrier of *qi*, especially the *qi* outside the vessels that must attach itself to body fluids in order to flow in the body. Loss of body fluids would inevitably lead to loss of *qi*.

13　Body fluids generate *qi*. Body fluids, just like blood, can promote the production of *qi* and transform into blood to nourish the viscera so as to maintain sufficiency of *qi* in the viscera and the whole body.

III. Relationships Between Blood and Body Fluid(s)

14　Blood and body fluids are both liquid substance with the function of nourishing and moistening the viscera and tissues. Compared with *qi*, blood and body fluid pertain to *yin*. This relationships between them can be generalized as "sharing the same origin".

15　Physiologically, blood and body fluids are both generated from food nutrients and can supplement and transform into each other. Pathologically, blood and body fluids can affect each other. For example, patients with excessive bleeding usually have symptoms of dry mouth, dry throat, scanty urine, and dry skin due to deficiency of body fluids. Clinically, patients with severe loss of blood should avoid diaphoresis and **diuresis** because profuse sweating consumes body fluids and further **aggravates** the deficiency of blood. Patients with severe loss of body fluids caused by severe sweating, vomiting or **diarrhea** should not be treated by blood consuming therapy to avoid further damage to body fluids. (958 words)

phlegm /flem/　*n*. 痰,黏液

bladder /ˈblædə/　*n*. 膀胱,囊状物

diuresis /ˌdaɪjʊ(ə)ˈriːsɪs/　*n*. 利尿,多尿

aggravate /ˈæɡrəveɪt/　*vt*. 加重,使恶化

diarrhea /ˌdaɪəˈrɪə/　*n*. 腹泻,痢疾

Notes：

1.　*Qi* pertains to *yang* while blood to *yin*. 气属阳,血属阴。

2.　The relationships between *qi* and blood are usually generalized as that "*qi* is the commander of blood and blood is the mother of *qi*". 气血关系通常被概括为"气为血之帅,血为气之母"。

3. food nutrients 水谷精微

4. visceral *qi* 脏腑之气

5. stagnation of *qi* 亦为 *qi* stagnation, 气滞

6. stasis of blood 亦为 blood stasis, 血瘀

7. If *qi* fails to propel or stagnates, it will lead to retarded blood circulation or blood stasis. 气的推动功能失司或气滞,将导致血行受阻或血瘀。

8. *Qi* commands blood to circulate inside vessels to avoid bleeding. 气统血,使血液在血脉里运行而不妄行。

9. *qi* deficiency 气虚

10. Blood carries *qi*. 血载气。

11. Sufficient *qi* of the spleen and stomach with prosperous *qi* transformation can generate sufficient body fluids, while deficient *qi* of the spleen and stomach with hypoactive *qi* transformation will lead to disorder of body fluids in generation, resulting in deficiency of body fluids. 脾胃之气旺盛,气化有力,则可生成充足的津液;脾胃之气亏虚,气化衰弱,则津液生成失常,最终导致津液不足。

12. The relationships between them can be generalized as "sharing the same origin". 它们之间的关系可以概括为"津血同源"。

13. Physiologically, blood and body fluids are both generated from food nutrients and can supplement and transform into each other. 生理上,血和津液都由水谷精微化生而来。它们可以相互补充,相互转化。

14. For example, patients with excessive bleeding usually have symptoms of dry mouth, dry throat, scanty urine, and dry skin due to deficiency of body fluids. 例如,患者流血过多(临床上)常表现为口干咽燥、尿液稀少、皮肤干燥等津液不足的症状。

15. Clinically, patients with severe loss of blood should avoid diaphoresis and diuresis because profuse sweating consumes body fluids and further aggravates the deficiency of blood; and patients with severe loss of body fluids caused by severe sweating or vomiting or diarrhea should not be treated by blood consuming therapy to avoid further damage to body fluids. 临床上,失血过多的患者应尽量避免发汗和利尿,因为大量出汗会耗损津液,加重血虚症状;而因出汗、呕吐或腹泻严重,导致津液大量损耗的患者则不宜再使用耗血疗法,以免加重津液损耗。

Task One   Reading Comprehension

1. Which of the following statements is **NOT** true according to TCM?

   A. Qi, blood and body fluids are different in nature.

   B. Qi, blood and body fluids act upon each other.

   C. Qi, blood and body fluids share the same origin.

   D. Qi, blood and body fluids are the same thing in function.

2. According to TCM theory, why do we call ying *qi* (营气) the nutrient or nutritive *qi*?

A. Because nutritive *qi* nourishes visceral *qi*.

B. Because nutritive *qi* can be transformed into blood when necessary.

C. Because nutritive *qi* protects our human body from exogenous pathogenic factors.

D. Because nutritive *qi* provides the Zang-Fu organs with nutrients.

3. According to TCM theory, blood circulation depends on the followings EXCEPT _____.

A. the driving force of the heart *qi*

B. the lung *qi*'s assistance of the heart in propelling blood to circulate inside the vessels

C. the stomach *qi*'s controlling function

D. the liver *qi*'s maintenance of smoothness of the blood circulation

4. According to TCM theory, the disordered distribution of body fluids is often manifested by _____.

A. edema   B. fluid retention

C. phlegm   D. all of the above

5. When we say blood and body fluids share the same origin, we do **NOT** mean _____.

A. blood and body fluids are both generated from food nutrients

B. severe loss of body fluids often leads to deficiency of *qi* and blood

C. profuse sweating consumes both body fluids and blood

D. blood and body fluids supplement and transform into each other

Task Two　Vocabulary

1. Directions: Complete the following phrases respectively according to its corresponding meaning or equivalent in Chinese within the brackets.

1) blood _____ (属) to *yin*

2) blood _____ (主) moisture and nourishment

3) *qi* _____ (气滞)

4) *qi* _____ (气化)

5) blood _____ (血瘀)

6) activating blood and _____ (化瘀)

7) promoting blood _____ (生成)

8) mutually _____ (影响)

9) _____ (充盈) of blood and *qi*

10) _____ (亏虚) of blood and *qi*

11) _____ (受阻的) blood circulation

12) *qi* failing to _____ blood (统血)

13) _____ (脏) *qi*

14) _____ (有力的) *qi* transformation

15) _____ (减退的) *qi* transformation

16) _____ (失调) of body fluids

17) fluid _____ (潴留)

18) _____（痰）and dampness

19) *qi* transformation of _____（膀胱）

20) _____ sweating（发汗）to release superficies

2. Fill in the blanks with the words from the box and change the form when necessary.

supplement	disperse	prosperous	bladder	phlegm
aggravate	stagnation	nutritive	generate	diaphoresis
sufficient	retard	hyperactive	diuresis	diarrhea

1) Her mother, a single parent, works in a restaurant and relies on tips to _____ wages.

2) On the one hand, wood _____ fire; on the other, it restrains earth.

3) Is personal protection equipment for medical personnel being provided in _____ quantities?

4) The _____ arguments still stand and I would not make a habit of eating lots of white bread.

5) By the 1980s and '90s, health insurance was becoming prohibitively costly, and wages were starting to _____ .

6) While the condition varies in severity, about three-quarters of people with autism are classed, in the official language of psychiatrists（精神病学家）, as mentally _____ .

7) "The rise of a strong, _____ China can be a source of strength for the community of nations," Mr Obama said.

8) The dark cloud of the financial crisis will _____ . Let us work together for a more splendid future.

9) Studies with functional magnetic resonance imaging（FMRI,功能性磁共振成像）show that people with anxiety disorders and those with mood disorders share a _____ response of the brain's amygdala region to negative emotion and aversion.

10) Cadmium（镉）is highly toxic, builds up in the body, and can cause stomach pains, vomiting and _____ .

11) Bunker _____ an old injury in her ribs, while Thompson sprained his neck and upper back.

12) When diagnosis is clear, active transfusion（输血,输液）, _____ , promoting uric acid excretion, hemodialysis（血液透析）and chemical therapy can improve prognosis.

13) My voice is like sandpaper, I cough up gobs（凝块）of _____ , and my liver feels like a sandbag.

14) I was overwhelmed with excitement, and became acutely aware of my own tachycardia（心跳过速）and _____ .

15) Unfortunately, no effective gall _____ plug has been developed despite considerable research in this field.

Task Three　Writing

Please rewrite the text in a form of abstract（about 150 words）

Terminology

Basic Terminology of Qi, Blood, Body fluids and Essence

Terminology	WHO	WFCMS
精气学说	essential *qi* theory	theory of essential *qi*
先天之精	innate essence	innate essence
后天之精	acquired essence	acquired essence
元气	source *qi*	original *qi*
宗气	ancestral *qi*	pectoral *qi*
卫气	defense *qi*	defense *qi*
营气	nutrient *qi*	nutrient *qi*
中气	middle *qi*	middle *qi*
气机	*qi* movement	*qi* movement/ transformation
营血	nutrient and blood	nutrient-blood
津液	fluid and humor	body fluids
津脱	fluid collapse	fluid collapse
津枯血燥	fluid consumption and blood dryness	fluid exhaustion and blood dryness
津血同源	homogeny of fluid and blood	fluid and blood from same source
营卫	nutrient and defense	nutrient-defense
膀胱	bladder	Bladder; CO (9); bladder (pangguang)
大汗	profuse sweating	profuse sweating
卫分	defense aspect	defense aspect
气分	*qi* aspect	*qi* aspect
营分	nutrient aspect	nutrient aspect
营卫不和	nutrient-defense disharmony	disharmony between nutrient and defensive *qi*
气不摄血	*qi* deficiency failing to control blood	failure of *qi* to control blood
气虚血瘀	*qi* deficiency with blood stasis	*qi* deficiency and blood stasis
气滞血瘀	blood stasis due to *qi* stagnation	*qi* stagnation and blood stasis
气滞	*qi* stagnation	*qi* stagnation
气闭	*qi* block	*qi* block
气脱	*qi* collapse	*qi* collapse
利水渗湿	induce diuresis to drain dampness	promoting urination and draining dampness
活血化瘀	activate blood and resolve stasis	activating blood and resolving stasis

continued

Terminology	WHO	WFCMS
补气	tonify *qi*	tonifying *qi*
蓄血证	blood amassment pattern/syndrome	blood accumulation syndrome/pattern
水生木	water engenders wood	water generating wood
血海	sea of blood	SP 10 (Xuehai); the sea of blood
气化不利	inhibited *qi* transformation	disturbance of *qi* transformation
痰蒙心包	phlegm clouding the pericardium	phlegm clouding pericardium
肝气不疏	constrained liver *qi*	constraining of liver *qi*

本书配套数字教学资源

微信扫描二维码，加入中医英语
读者交流圈，获取配套教学视
频、学习课件、课后习题和沟通交
流平台等板块内容，夯实基础知识

If yang fails to dominate over yin, *qi* from the Five Zang-Organs will be in disorder, blocking the nine orifices.

阳不胜其阴,则五脏气争,九窍不通①。

Unit 5　Etiology and pathogenesis

Warming-up

Before you listen (Watch)

In this section you will hear a short passage about "Six Evils". The following words and phrases may be of help.

mechanics /məˈkænɪks/	*n*.	运作方式
perspective /pəˈspektɪv/	*n*.	观点
resilient /rɪˈzɪlɪənt/	*adj*.	能复原的
dramatic /drəˈmætɪk/	*adj*.	急剧的
pore /pɔː(r)/	*n*.	毛孔
perspire /pəˈspaɪə(r)/	*vi*.	流汗

While you listen(Watch)

Listen to the passage carefully and fill in each of the blanks marked from 1) to 10) according to what you have heard.

So the six evils, as I will get to in the moment, describe basically the various external 1) _____ , maybe more specifically, environmentally, or even weather-induced stressors. So these are things that occur in nature, that usually start externally that 2) _____ the body. It can cause internal imbalances. So in simpler terms, the six evils pretty much refer to external stressors that are caused by the environment essentially that affect the body 3) _____ . And as you'll see once we get into the six evils, these are all found in nature. And because the human body is a piece of nature and it carries the same components and 4) _____ as nature does, when the body

---

① 《素问·四气调神大论篇》,李照国译。

becomes imbalanced in terms of Chinese medicine, there is often one of the six evils going out of hand, so in another word the way the six evils causing 5) _____ in the body is basically by excess. So any one of these things are not necessarily 6) _____ evil, it's just dependent upon a person's constitution, and whether or not one of these evils is dramatic, and it is very excessive, or just the sensitivity that person might have to that particular evil.

So getting right into the six evils. The first evil is referred to as 7) _____ evil. So this isn't to say that you will get sick just by being exposed to wind or going out on a windy day. However, wind in Chinese medicine can affect the skin predominantly, so the wind can attack the skin by basically going to the pores and how wind can attribute to a disease or a 8) _____ like infection or some sort of imbalance in the body is that wind can set the stage for other imbalances. So in the case of extreme wind, wind can attack the pores and leave the pores and the skin open to 9) _____. And external pathogens and various things can be occurring in the external environment. However, if your body is generally in 10) _____ and good health, and it is not under too much stress, you probably can be pretty resilient to most conditions with the wind, wind isn't going to be the most extreme evil.

After you listen(Watch)

Please discuss with your partner the following questions and give your presentation to the class.

1) What do the six evils describe according to the speaker?
2) What are the possible factors of whether one will be ill or not after being exposed to the six evils?
3) What will wind evil affect predominantly in the human body?
4) What part of the body is affected in a wind invasion?

Reading

 Text A

BEFORE CLASS

1. **Quest for Definition**

Directions: Explore online the definitions of the following terms from Text A and prepare a unique one-minute oral presentation for your class.

1) etiology
2) nine orifices
3) six excesses
4) seven emotions
5) static blood

2. Text-based Activities

Directions: Read carefully the part of Text A that corresponds to your task, and then prepare a unique one-minute oral presentation for your class.

PERFORMANCE IN CLASS

Your Task

1) When does a disease usually occur according to TCM?

2) What do pathogenic factors involve as described in the text?

3) Please describe briefly the three classifications of pathogenic factors in the book entitled *Jingui Yaolue* (*Synopsis of Golden Chamber*).

4) If a person often has cold and uncooked food, what symptoms will it usually bring on?

5) What will lead to static blood?

Etiology

1   TCM holds that the body keeps a dynamic equilibrium between the internal and external environments as well between as the viscera and the tissues①. Such a dynamic equilibrium maintains the normal physiological activities of the body. If the dynamic equilibrium is damaged and cannot be restored immediately, it will lead to disease.

2   The cause of disease, or etiology, refers to the factors that damage the dynamic equilibrium and result in disease. Pathogenic factors are various, and can include abnormal changes of weather, **pestilence**, mental stimulation, improper diet, overstrain, **trauma** due to heavy load, injury caused by falling, **incised** wound and insect or animal bites, etc.② During the course of a disease, the cause and effect are often interacting with each other③. Take phlegm, retained fluid and static blood for example. They are the pathological substances caused by dysfunction of the viscera, *qi* and blood on the one hand, and the pathogenic factors that lead to diseases on the other.

3   In the *Nei Jing*, pathogenic factors were classified into two major categories, namely *yin* and *yang*. In the *Su Wen*, for example, it says the pathogenic factors originate either from the *yin*

---

①   TCM holds that the body keeps a dynamic equilibrium between the internal and external environments as well as the viscera and the tissues: 中医学认为,人体各脏腑组织之间,以及人体与外界环境之间维持着相对的动态平衡。

②   Pathogenic factors are various, and can include abnormal changes of weather, pestilence, mental stimulation, improper diet, overstrain, trauma due to heavy load, injury caused by falling, incised wound and insect or animal bites, etc.: 病邪多种多样,如气候的异常、疫病的传染、精神刺激、饮食劳倦、持重努伤、跌仆金刃外伤,以及虫兽所伤等。

③   During the course of a disease, the cause and effect are often interacting with each other: 在疾病过程中,原因和结果是相互作用着的。

aspect or from the *yang* aspect. Those from the *yang* aspect are caused by wind, rain, cold and summer-heat, while those from the *yin* aspect are caused by improper diet and living conditions, sexual overindulgence and emotional changes. In the Eastern Han Dynasty, Zhang Zhongjing summarized pathogenic factors into three kinds in his book entitled *Jingui Yaolue* (*Synopsis of the Golden Chamber*). "Diseases are exclusively caused by three kinds of pathogenic factors. The first group is endogenous ones caused by invasion of exogenous pathogenic factors into the viscera from the meridians; the second group is diseases attacking the skin and stagnating the vessels that connect the four limbs and nine orifices; and the third group is the injuries caused by sexual overindulgence, incised wounds, and insect and animal bites.①" In the Song Dynasty, Chen Wuze②. also summarized the causes of diseases into three categories, namely; "internal causes, external causes and causes neither internal nor external".

4   Abnormal changes of weather, known as six excesses, are the most commonly encountered exogenous pathogenic factors, including wind, cold, summer-heat, dampness, dryness and fire. Under normal conditions, they are six climatic changes indispensable to the growth of all living things in nature. However, when they are excessive or insufficient, or when they do not take place at the appropriate time, or when the body resistance is too weak to adapt to the climatic changes, these six climatic changes will become pathogenic factors. Sometimes **dysfunction** of the viscera brings on the symptoms similar to the ones caused by invasion of external wind, cold, dampness, dryness and fire. In order to distinguish them from the six external pathogenic factors, they are called "five internal excesses", namely internal wind, internal cold, internal dampness, internal dryness and internal fire③.

5   Pestilence is a kind of **fulminating** infectious pathogenic factors. Diseases caused by pestilence include many of the infectious and epidemic diseases in modern medicine, such as pestilent dysentery, **diphtheria**, smallpox, **cholera** and **plague**. The occurrence and spread of pestilence are related to a number of factors, such as climate, environment, diet, lack of timely prevention and isolation.

6   Emotions are normal reactions of the body and mind to the external environment and are usually classified into seven kinds, including joy, anger, anxiety, thought, sorrow, fear and

---

①   Diseases are exclusively caused by three kinds of pathogenic factors. The first group is endogenous ones caused by invasion of exogenous pathogenic factors into the viscera from the meridians; the second group is the ones attacking the skin and stagnating the vessels that connect the four limbs and nine orifices; and the third group is the injuries caused by sexual overindulgence, incised wound and insect and animal bites：千般疢难，不越三条，一者，经络受邪，入脏腑，为内所因也；二者，四肢九窍，血脉相传，壅塞不通，为外皮肤所中也；三者，房室、金刃、虫兽所伤。nine orifices：九窍指人体的两眼、两耳、两鼻孔、口、前阴尿道和后阴肛门。《素问·生气通天论篇》："天地之间，六合之内，其气九州、九窍、五藏、十二节，皆通乎天气。"

②   Chen Wuze：陈无择(1131—1189 年)，宋代处州青田(今浙江青田县人)。他的主要著作《三因极一病证方论》继承、发展了《黄帝内经》《伤寒杂病论》等的病因学理论，创立了病因分类的"三因学说"。

③   In order to distinguish them from the six external pathogenic factors, they are called "five internal excesses", namely internal wind, internal cold, internal dampness, internal dryness and internal fire：为了将其与六邪区分开来，它们被称为"内生五邪"，即内风、内寒、内湿、内燥、内火。

fright. Under normal conditions, the seven emotions will not cause disease. However, sudden, strong and continuous emotional stimulation will lead to disorder of visceral *yin* and *yang* as well as *qi* and blood, resulting in diseases. Since abnormal change of emotions is the major factor causing internal problems, it is termed "internal injury due to seven emotions"①. The disorder of the seven emotions usually directly affects the relevant viscera because of the close relationship between the viscera and emotions. That is why the *Su Wen* states that "excessive anger damages the liver"; "excessive joy damages the heart"; "excessive thought damages the spleen"; "excessive anxiety damages the lung"; "excessive fright or fear damages the kidney". It is also said that "excessive anger drives *qi* to flow upward"; "excessive joy makes *qi* **sluggish**"; "excessive sorrow consumes *qi*"; "excessive fear drives *qi* to flow downward"; "excessive fright disorders *qi*"; "excessive thought stagnates *qi*"②.

7　Diet provides nourishment for the body and maintains the activities of life. However, improper diet or imbalanced diet frequently leads to diseases. When taken into the body, food depends on the spleen and stomach to digest. Improper diet will affect the physiological functions of the spleen and stomach, eventually resulting in the accumulation of dampness, production of phlegm, transformation of heat or other pathological changes. The commonly encountered diseases caused by improper diet are disorders of gastrointestinal tract, such as abdominal pain, vomiting, diarrhea and dysentery, or parasitic diseases, such as ascariasis, oxyuriasis and taeniasis. Predilection for one of the flavors will also bring on a number of problems. For instance, **predilection** for cold and uncooked food impairs the spleen and the stomach *yang* and leads to internal cold and dampness that will eventually result in abdominal pain and diarrhea. Predilection for acrid, warm, dry and hot food may accumulate heat in the intestines and stomach, bringing on such symptoms as thirst, abdominal distension and pain, constipation and **hemorrhoids**.

8　Phlegm and fluid retention are another pair of pathogenic factors in TCM, both of which are the pathological substances produced during the course of a disease. The former is thick and the latter is thin. "Phlegm" not only refers to sputum **expectorated** from the throat, but also includes **scrofula**, **nodules** and the thick liquid substance retained or stagnated in the viscera and meridians③. Fluid retention refers to fluid that is retained in the local regions. Phlegm usually results in asthmatic cough with expectoration if it is retained in the lung; chest distress and palpitation if it is stagnated in the heart; unconsciousness and **dementia** if it confuses the mind; mania if it transforms into fire and disturbs the heart; nausea, vomiting and stomach fullness if it is retained in the

---

①　Since abnormal change of emotions is the major factor causing internal problems, it is termed "internal injury due to seven emotions": 由于情志异常是造成内伤病的主要原因,所以称为"内伤七情"。

②　"excessive anger drives *qi* to flow upward"; "excessive joy makes *qi* sluggish"; "excessive sorrow consumes *qi*"; "excessive fear drives *qi* to flow downward"; "excessive fright disorders *qi*" and "excessive thought stagnates *qi*":"怒则气上;喜则气缓;悲则气消;恐则气下;惊则气乱;思则气结。"

③　"Phlegm" not only refers to sputum expectorated from the throat, but also includes scrofula, nodules and the thick liquid substance retained or stagnated in the viscera and meridians:"痰"不仅仅指从喉咙咯吐出来的痰,也包括瘰疬、痰核和停滞在脏腑经络等组织中而未被排出的痰液。

stomach; and scrofula, numbness of limbs or paralysis if it is retained in the meridians, tendons and bones; vertigo if it attacks the head; obstructive sensation in the throat if it stagnates in the throat. Fluid retention in the gastrointestinal tract often leads to intestinal gurgling if it is retained in the intestines; chest and **hypochondriac** distension and fullness as well as pain during cough if it is retained in the chest and hypochondria; chest distress, cough, dyspnea and inability to lie flat if it is retained in the chest and diaphragm; **subcutaneous** edema, **anhidrosis** and body pain if it is retained in the skin.

9   Stasis of blood is also one of the commonly encountered pathogenic factors. Stasis of blood can be caused either by deficiency and stagnation of qi, blood cold and blood heat, or by internal and external injury and extravasations of blood due to blood heat[①]. Blood stasis frequently causes **palpitation**, chest distress, heart pain and cyanotic nails and lips if it is retained in the heart; chest pain and **hemoptysis** if it is retained in the lung; **hematemesis** and black feces if it is retained in the intestines and stomach; hypochondriac pain and mass if it is retained in the liver; mania if it attacks the heart; lower abdominal pain, irregular menstruation, **dysmenorrhea**, **amenorrhea**, purplish color of menstruation with blood clot or profuse uterine bleeding if it is retained in the uterus; local swelling, pain and **cyanosis** if it is retained in the limbs and muscles. (1,302 words)

New Words and Expressions

pestilence /'pestɪləns/ *n*. a disease that causes death and spreads quickly to large numbers of people, especially bubonic plague 瘟疫(尤指腺鼠疫)

trauma /'trɔːmə/ *n*. an injury 损伤, 外伤

incise /ɪn'saɪz/ *vt*. to cut words, designs, etc. into a surface (在表面)雕, 刻; 切入

dysfunction /dɪs'fʌŋkʃn/ *n*. abnormality in the operation of a specified bodily organ or system 机能 (功能)障碍

fulminating /'fʌlmɪneɪtɪŋ/ *adj*. (of a disease or symptom) developing suddenly and severely 暴发性的

diphtheria /dɪf'θɪərɪə/ *n*. 白喉

cholera /'kɒlərə/ *n*. 霍乱

plague /pleɪg/ *n*. an attack of disease causing death and spreading quickly to a large number of people 瘟疫; 传染病; 疫病

sluggish /'slʌgɪʃ/ *adj*. slow-moving; not very active or quick 行动迟缓的; 不活泼的; 缓慢的

gastrointestinal /ˌgæstrəʊɪn'testɪnl/ *adj*. of the stomach and intestine 胃肠的

parasitic /ˌpærə'sɪtɪk/ *adj*. of parasite 寄生的

ascariasis /ˌæskə'raɪəsɪs/ *n*. 蛔虫病

oxyuriasis /ˌɒksɪjʊə'raɪəsɪs/ *n*. 蛲虫病

---

①   Static blood can be caused either by deficiency and stagnation of qi, blood cold and blood heat, or by internal and external injury and extravasations of blood due to blood heat: 瘀血或由气虚、气滞、血寒、血热等原因所造成, 或由内外伤或血热妄行等原因所引起。

taeniasis /tiːˈnaɪəsɪs/ *n.* 绦虫病

predilection /ˌpriːdɪˈlekʃn/ *n.* special preference for something 偏爱, 嗜好

hemorrhoid /ˈhemərɔɪd/ *n.* a swollen blood vessel at the anus 痔疮

expectorate /ɪkˈspektəreɪt/ *v.* to force liquid from the mouth; spit 吐出(痰)

scrofula /ˈskrɒfjʊlə/ *n.* a form of tuberculosis affecting the lymph nodes, especially of the neck 淋巴结核

nodule /ˈnɒdjuːl/ *n.* a small knot like protuberance 小节结

hypochondriac /ˌhaɪpəˈkɒndrɪæk/ *adj.* 季肋的

subcutaneous /ˌsʌbkjuˈteɪnɪəs/ *adj.* beneath the skin 皮下的

dementia /dɪˈmenʃə/ *n.* decay of the mind, especially leading to madness 痴呆

anhidrosis /ˌænhaɪˈdrəʊsɪs/ *n.* no sweating 无汗(症)

palpitation /pælpɪˈteɪʃ(ə)n/ *n.* irregular, rapid beating or pulsation of the heart 心悸

hematemesis /ˌhiːməˈtemɪsɪs/ *n.* vomiting blood 吐血, 咯血

hemoptysis /hɪˈmɒptɪsɪs/ *n.* coughing up blood from the respiratory tract 咳血; 咯血

dysmenorrhea /ˌdɪsmenəˈrɪə/ *n.* painful menstruation, typically involving abdominal cramps 痛经

amenorrhea /eɪˌmenəˈriːə/ *n.* an abnormal absence of menstruation 闭经

cyanosis /saɪəˈnəʊsɪs/ *n.* a bluish discoloration of the skin due to poor circulation or inadequate oxygenation of the blood 发绀, 青紫

FOLLOW-UP ACTIVITIES

Task One   Comprehension Check

1. Questions for Discussion

1) How many pathogenic factors are mentioned in the text? What are they?

2) What are the major different classifications of pathogenic factors in TCM mentioned in the text?

3) How do emotions bring on diseases?

4) What is the relationship between diet and health?

2. Chart Completion

TCM'S THEORY ABOUT FUNCTION OF DYNAMIC EQUILIBRIUM:

INTRODUCTION: (para. 1)
According to Traditional Chinese Medicine (TCM), a dynamic equilibrium maintains the normal 1) _____ of the body. If the dynamic equilibrium is damaged and not restored immediately, a disease tends to occur.

VARIOUS PATHOGEIC FACTORS THAT DAMAGE DYNAMIC FACTORS AND THEIR CLASSIFICATIONS IN DIFFERENT TCM SOURCES: (para. 2 - 3)
- *Huangdi Neijing*, the earliest and greatest medical classic extant in China, classified pathogenic factors into two categories, namely 2) _____.

- *Jinggui Yaolue* by Zhang Zhongjing in the Eastern Han Dynasty divided pathogenic factors into three groups. The first group involves endogenous ones caused by 3) _____ ____ pathogenic factors into the viscera from the meridians; the second group includes the ones attacking the skin and stagnating the vessels that 4) _____ ; the third group is the injuries resulting from 5) _____ .
- Chen Wuze in the Song Dynasty summarized the causes into three categories, that is, internal causes, external causes and causes 6) _____ .

ILLUSTRATION OF SIX PATHOGENIC FACTORS: (para. 4 – 9)

- Abnormal changes of weather such as wind, cold, summer-heat, dampness, dryness and fire will become pathogenic factors leading to diseases when they are 7) _____ or when they don't take place 8) _____ .
- Pestilence, a kind of fulminating infectious pathogenic factors, results from a number of causes such as climate, environment and lack of 9) _____ , etc.
- Emotions, under normal conditions, will not cause diseases, but when the emotional stimulation is 10) _____ , it will bring on diseases.
- Diet often leads to diseases if it is 11) _____ . For example, if a person prefers cold and uncooked food, it tends to result in the occurrence of 12) _____ .
- Phlegm and fluid retention are the pathological substances produced during the 13) _____ _____ . The former includes not only sputum expectorated from the throat, but also scrofula, nodules and the thick liquid substance retained or stagnated in the 14) _____ _____ . The latter refers to fluid retained in the 15) _____ .
- Static blood, one of the commonly encountered pathogenic factors, results either from 16) _____ of qi, blood cold and blood heat, or from internal and external injury and extravasations of blood due to blood heat.

Task Two   Vocabulary

1. **Directions**: Complete the following phrases respectively according to its corresponding meaning or equivalent in Chinese within the brackets.

1) the _____ (发生) of disease

2) _____ (不正常的) changes of weather

3) _____ (寄生的) diseases

4) four limbs and nine _____ (孔窍)

5) _____ (适应) the climatic changes

6) _____ (没有规律的) menstruation

7) take static blood _____ (为例)

8) _____ (不正常的) changes of weather

9) _____ (起源于) the y*in* aspect

10) _____ (不恰当的) diet

11) _____ (内外的) injury

12) _____(外部的) environment

13) _____(影响) the relevant viscera

14) _____(过度的) anger or joy

15) result in the _____(累积) of dampness

16) _____(偏爱) for uncooked food

17) continuous emotional _____(刺激)

18) bring on the _____(症状)

19) the normal _____(生理学的) activities

20) lead to the _____(发生) of disease

21) trauma _____(由于) heavy load

22) _____(功能障碍) of the viscera

23) _____(内生性的) causes

24) _____(不平衡的) diet

25) _____(病理学的) substances

26) result in _____(腹部的) pain

27) _____(不足) and stagnation of *qi*

28) disorders of_____(胃肠的) tract

29) _____(不规律的) menstruation

30) lack of _____(及时的) prevention and isolation

2. Match the following words with their proper meanings.

Column I	Column II
1) occurrence	a. a state of balance, especially between opposing forces or influences
2) profuse	b. only; solely
3) dysfunction	c. relating to breathing with a whistling sound
4) asthmatic	d. not moving, changing or developing
5) etiology	e. something that happens or exists
6) retain	f. any infectious disease that spreads quickly and kills a lot of people
7) predilection	g. abnormality in the operation of a specified bodily organ or system
8) transform	h. food that is needed to stay alive, grow and stay healthy
9) restore	i. produced in large amounts
10) exclusively	j. preference; liking
11) expectorate	k. to bring sb/ sth back to a former condition, place or position
12) static	l. the cause of a disease
13) nourishment	m. to change the form of sth
14) equilibrium	n. to continue to hold or contain
15) pestilence	o. to cough and make phlegm come up from your lungs into your mouth so you can spit it out

3. Fill in the blanks with the words from the box and change the form when necessary.

dynamic	maintain	occurrence	palpitation	abnormal
dementia	improper	connect	encounter	reaction
distinguish	plague	namely	parasitic	external

1) So again, take your mind back to a week ago when you had this dream and see if you can _____ any of the above to what was going on in your life as well as in your mind.

2) Panicking and focusing on our nightmares will not help us get through the coronavirus _____.

3) Detecting signs of life elsewhere will not be easy, but it may well _____ in my lifetime, if not during the next decade.

4) What matters most are what real consumers spend their money on and how they _____ to the prices of those things.

5) The Redondo Beach site provides assisted living for seniors and memory care to those with Alzheimer's disease and other forms of _____.

6) He said there is no alternative for him but to _____ order under any circumstances.

7) In life we should be striving for _____ balance, not a static one.

8) These behaviors are known to benefit health in many other ways, _____ lowering the risk of obesity, diabetes and heart disease and improving mood.

9) We think we may have an almost complete understanding of the set of _____ genes which drive this cancer.

10) Media reports said he suffered chest pain or heart _____.

11) Of course, we all _____ problems and obstacles every day, but most of them are trivial compared with the problems many people experience.

12) It means that you have to _____ between what you see and what you believe.

13) Long-term storage and _____ disposal of this material may result in dioxin (二噁英) release into the environment and the contamination of human and animal food supplies.

14) You can work with your brainwaves through meditation or by using a(n) _____ stimulus such as brainwave audios.

15) About two billion of the world's poorest people are infected with _____ worms.

Task Three   Translation

1. Translate the following medical expressions into English

1) 致病因素
2) 四肢九窍
3) 动态平衡
4) 持重努伤
5) 瘀血
6) 气候异常
7) 虫兽所伤
8) 精神刺激
9) 怒则气上
10) 内伤七情

11）内生五邪   12）寒生食物

13）悲则气消   14）气血障碍

15）腹部疼痛   16）胃肠道

17）纵欲   18）爆发性传染病

19）月经不调   20）内脏和组织

2. Translate the following sentences into Chinese or English

1) TCM maintains that human body keeps a dynamic balance between the internal and external environments. If the dynamic balance is damaged and not restored immediately, diseases often occur.

2) The TCM classic book entitled *Nei Jing* classifies pathogenic factors into two categories, namely *yin* and *yang*.

3) Sudden, strong and continuous emotional stimulation will lead to disorder of visceral *yin* and *yang* as well as *qi* and blood, consequently bringing on diseases.

4) Improper diet will affect the physiological functions of the spleen and stomach, eventually resulting in the accumulation of dampness, production of phlegm, transformation of heat or other pathological changes.

5) Static blood can be caused either by deficiency and stagnation of *qi*, blood cold and blood heat, or by internal and external injury and extravasations of blood due to blood heat.

6) 七情内伤直接影响相应的内脏，使脏腑气机逆乱，气血失调，导致种种疾病的发生。

7) 破坏人体相对动态平衡状态而引起疾病的原因就是病因。

8) 饮食不节主要是损伤脾胃，导致脾胃功能失常。

9) 六淫是风、寒、暑、湿、燥、火六种外感病邪的统称。

10) 在宋代，陈无择将病因归纳为三类，即内因、外因、不内外因。

3. Translate the following passage into English

  病因学的定义是造成疾病的各种原因。在中医看来，病因主要有六淫、疫气、七情、饮食不节、劳逸失度、外伤、痰饮、瘀血等。何谓病机？病机指的是疾病发生、发展和转归的机制。疾病的发生、发展和转归与人体的正气和病邪特性密切相关。

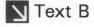 Text B

Pathogenesis

1 Pathogenesis refers to the **mechanism** involved in the occurrence, progress and changes of disease that are closely related to the constitution of the patient and the nature of pathogenic factors.

mechanism /ˈmekənɪzəm/ *n*.（行为的）机制

2 When pathogenic factors attack the body, healthy *qi* in the

body naturally fights against them. Such a struggle between healthy *qi* and pathogenic factors damages the relative equilibrium between *yin* and *yang* in the body, leads to dysfunction of the viscera and meridians, or results in disturbance of *qi* and blood, which consequently brings on various local or general pathological changes. Although diseases vary and clinical manifestations are complicated, pathogenesis, in general, involves only such factors as exuberance and decline of healthy *qi* and pathogenic factors, disharmony between *yin* and *yang*, disorder of *qi* and blood as well as dysfunction of the viscera and meridians.

3　During the course of a disease, the conditions of healthy *qi* and pathogenic factors are not fixed, but interact with each other and change constantly. Generally speaking, **superabundance** of healthy *qi* will reduce pathogenic factors and exuberance of pathogenic factors will consume healthy *qi* accordingly. The increase or decrease of healthy *qi* and pathogenic factors are responsible for the deficiency and excess changes of diseases.

4　Deficiency mainly refers to insufficiency of healthy *qi*, indicating hypofunction of *qi*, blood, body fluid, meridians and viscera. In this case the healthy *qi* is difficult to launch an intense struggle against pathogenic factors and eventually leads to a deficiency syndrome. The clinical manifestations of deficiency syndrome are spiritual and physical **lassitude**, **lusterless** complexion, palpitation, shortness of breath, **spontaneous** sweating, night sweating, feverish sensation over five centers (palms, soles and chest), or aversion to cold, cold limbs and weak pulse.

5　Excess mainly refers to superabundance of pathogenic factors, indicating that both the pathogenic factors and the body resistance are strong or the pathogenic factors are strong but the healthy *qi* is not weak. Under such a condition, the conflict between healthy *qi* and pathogenic factors is intense and brings on an excess syndrome. The clinical manifestations of excess syndrome are profuse phlegm, indigestion, accumulation of fluid and dampness, interior retention of blood stasis, high fever, mania, high and coarse voice, constipation, **dysuria** and powerful pulse.

6　Disharmony between *yin* and *yang* refers to the relative exuberance or **debilitation** of *yin* and *yang* or failure of *yin* to control *yang* or *yang* to control *yin* due to various pathogenic

exuberance /ɪɡˈzjuːbərəns/ *n.* 茂盛

superabundance /ˌsuːpərəˈbʌndəns/ *n.* 过多，多余

lassitude /ˈlæsɪtjuːd/ *n.* 无力；困乏；倦怠
lusterless /ˈlʌstəlɪs/ *adj.* 无光泽的
spontaneous /spɒnˈteɪnɪəs/ *adj.* 自然的；自发的(行为)
sole /səʊl/ *n.* 足底

dysuria /dɪsˈjʊərɪə/ *n.* 排尿困难

debilitation /dɪˌbɪlɪˈteɪʃən/ *n.* 虚弱

factors. The pathological changes of disharmony between *yin* and *yang* mainly include relative exuberance, relative debilitation, mutual consumption, mutual **repulsion** and depletion of *yin* and *yang*.

7　Relative exuberance of *yin* or *yang* mainly refers to excess syndrome because "exuberance of pathogenic factors leads to excess when pathogenic factors of *yang* nature invade the body, relative *yang* exuberance occurs with such symptoms as high fever, flushed face and red eyes, etc." The Su Wen states that *yang* exuberance causes exterior heat. When pathogenic factors of *yin* nature attack the body, relative *yin* exuberance occurs due to attack of cold dampness, excessive taking of uncooked and cold food, stagnation of cold in the middle energizer or internal exuberance of *yin* cold. The manifestations of relative *yin* exuberance are usually cold sensation of the body, cold limbs and a light-colored tongue.

8　Relative debilitation of *yin* or *yang* refers to deficiency syndrome because "loss of essence leads to deficiency". Relative debilitation of *yang* usually indicates deficient cold syndrome due to insufficiency of *yang* and relative exuberance of *yin* in the body. Relative debilitation of *yang* is mainly caused by congenital deficiency, or **postnatal malnutrition**, **endogenous** impairment due to overstrain, or consumption of *yang qi* due to prolonged illness. The usual symptoms caused by *yang* deficiency are fear of cold, cold limbs, a light-colored tongue, slow pulse, profuse and clear urine and diarrhea with indigested food. Relative debilitation of *yin* refers to a **morbid** state marked by relative exuberance of *yang* due to loss or consumption of essence, blood and body fluid and failure of *yin* to control *yang*. The various causes of relative decline of *yin* are pathogenic factors of *yang* nature impairing *yin*, fire transformed from extreme changes of emotions damaging *yin* and consumption of *yin* due to prolonged illness. The usual symptoms caused by relative debilitation of *yin* are feverish sensation over the five centers, bone-steaming, tidal fever, flushed cheeks, **emaciation**, night sweating, dry mouth and throat, a reddish tongue with scanty coating as well as thin, rapid and weak pulse.

9　Mutual consumption means that the deficiency of *yin* or *yang* affects the other, consequently bringing on dual deficiency of *yin*

repulsion /rɪˈpʌlʃn/ *n*. 厌恶，排斥

postnatal /ˌpəʊstˈneɪtl/ *adj*. 产后的；分娩后的；出生后的

malnutrition /ˌmælnjuˈtrɪʃn/ *n*. 营养不良

endogenous /enˈdɒdʒənəs/ *adj*. 内源的

morbid /ˈmɔːbɪd/ *adj*. 病态的

emaciation /ɪˌmeɪsɪˈeɪʃn/ *n*. 消瘦

and *yang*. *Yin* deficiency leading to *yang* deficiency is known as *yin* impairment affecting *yang* and *yang* deficiency resulting in *yin* deficiency is called *yang* impairment affecting *yin*. *Yin* impairment affecting *yang* refers to a morbid state marked by deficiency of both *yin* and *yang* resulting from *yin* deficiency due to loss of *yin* fluid that makes the production of *yang qi* deficient. For example, hyperactivity of liver *yang* is mainly caused by *yin* deficiency with *yang* hyperactivity. However, further development of such a pathological condition may consume kidney essence and impair kidney *yang*, eventually transforming into deficiency of both *yin* and *yang* due to the consumption of *yang* by *yin*. *Yang* impairment affecting *yin* refers to a morbid state marked by deficiency of both *yin* and *yang* resulting from *yang* deficiency that affects the production of *yin* fluid. For instance, edema is mainly caused by insufficiency of *yang qi*, dysfunction of *qi* transformation, disturbance of water metabolism and retention of fluid. However, further development of this pathological condition may transform into deficiency of both *yin* and *yang* due to the consumption of *yin* by *yang*, leading to such symptoms as emaciation, restlessness and even flaccidity.

edema /ɪˈdiːmə/ *n*. 水肿

flaccidity /flækˈsɪdɪtɪ/ *n*. 软弱;没气力

10   *Yin* and *yang* repulsion means that the extreme exuberance of either *yin* or *yang* stagnates inside and rejects the other, consequently bringing on complicated pathological phenomena such as true cold with false heat or true heat with false cold. Exuberant *yin* repelling *yang* means that interior exuberance of *yin* drives *yang* to float exteriorly, clinically leading to such false heat symptoms as flushed cheeks, dysphoric fever, thirst and large pulse. Exuberant *yang* repelling *yin* means that interior predominance of pathogenic heat stagnates *yang* and prevents it from reaching the limbs, clinically resulting in such false cold symptoms as deep cold sensation of the limbs and sunken pulse.

repel /rɪˈpel/ *v*. 排斥

11   *Yin* collapse or *yang* collapse refers to a critical state due to sudden and excessive loss of *yin* fluid or *yang qi*. *Yang* collapse means sudden depletion of *yang qi*, usually caused by exuberance of pathogenic factors and deficiency of healthy *qi*; or by frequent deficiency of *yang qi*, insufficiency of healthy *qi* and overstrain; or by improper use of emetic therapy and profuse sweating. *Yang* collapse in chronic and consumptive disease is usually due to serious exhaustion of *yang qi*. *Yin* collapse is frequently caused by

superabundance of pathogenic heat or prolonged retention of pathogenic heat, or other factors that scorches *yin* fluid, or excessively consumes *yin* fluid.

12　Besides, the disorders of *qi*, blood and body fluid, internal pathogenic substances (known as "five internal excess") as well as the dysfunction of meridians and viscera are also important factors responsible for various general or local pathological changes. (1,221 words)

Notes:

1. Such a struggle between healthy *qi* and pathogenic factors damages the relative equilibrium between *yin* and *yang* in the body, or leads to dysfunction of the viscera and meridians, or results in disturbance of *qi* and blood, which consequently brings on various local or general pathological changes. 本句中, healthy *qi* 指正气, pathogenic factor 指邪气。

2. Although diseases vary and clinical manifestations are complicated, the pathogenesis, in general, involves no more than such factors as exuberance and decline of healthy *qi* and pathogenic factors, disharmony between *yin* and *yang*, disorder of *qi* and blood as well as dysfunction of the viscera and meridians. 本句中, 主语 pathogenesis 和谓语 involves 之间插入了 in general。理解整个句子时可以对 in general 的位置按中文语序进行调换。

3. The clinical manifestations of excess syndrome are profuse phlegm, indigestion, accumulation of fluid and dampness, interior retention of blood stasis, high fever, mania, high and coarse voice, constipation, dysuria and powerful pulse, etc. 实证的临床表现是痰涎壅盛, 食积不化, 水湿泛滥, 瘀血内阻, 壮热, 狂躁, 声高气粗, 二便不通, 脉实有力等。

4. The pathological changes of disharmony between *yin* and *yang* mainly include relative exuberance, relative debilitation, mutual consumption, mutual repulsion and depletion of *yin* and *yang*. 阴阳失调的病理变化主要包括阴阳偏胜、阴阳偏衰、阴阳互损、阴阳格拒和阴阳亡失。注意偏胜、偏衰、互损、格据、亡失的英文表达。

5. Relative debilitation of *yin* or *yang* refers to deficiency syndrome because "loss of essence leads to deficiency". 本句中, loss of essence lead to deficiency 指的是"精气夺则虚"。

6. Relative debilitation of *yang* is mainly caused by congenital deficiency, or postnatal malnutrition and endogenous impairment due to overstrain, or consumption of *yang qi* due to prolonged illness. 本句中用 congenital deficiency 表示先天不足, 注意 congenital 所指的先天是病态情况, 故先天之精的"先天"不能用此词而需改用 prenatal 或 innate。

7. The various causes of relative decline of *yin* are pathogenic factors of *yang* nature impairing *yin*, fire transformed from extreme changes of emotions damaging *yin* and consumption of *yin* due to prolonged illness. 阴偏衰原因众多, 如阳邪伤阴, 五志过极, 化火伤阴, 久病伤阴。

8. The usual symptoms caused by relative debilitation of *yin* are feverish sensation over the five centers, bone-steaming, tidal fever, flushed cheeks, emaciation, night sweating, dry mouth and throat and reddish tongue with scanty coating as well as thin, rapid and weak pulse.注意本

句中 feverish sensation over the five centers, bone-steaming, tidal fever, flushed cheeks, emaciation, night sweating 分别指五心烦热、骨蒸、潮热、面赤、消瘦、盗汗。

9. *Yin* deficiency leading to *yang* deficiency is known as *yin* impairment affecting *yang*. 阴虚而导致阳虚称为阴损及阳。

10. *Yin* and *yang* repulsion means that the extreme exuberance of either *yin* or *yang* stagnates inside and rejects the other, consequently bringing on complicated pathological phenomena such as true cold with false heat or true heat with false cold. 阴阳格拒指阴或阳的一方偏盛至极,因而壅遏于内,将另一方排斥格拒于外,从而出现真寒假热或真热假寒的复杂病理现象。

11. Exuberant *yin* repelling *yang* means that interior exuberance of *yin* drives *yang* to float exteriorly, clinically leading to such false heat symptoms as flushed cheeks, dysphoric fever, thirst and large pulse. 阴盛格阳指阴寒之邪壅盛于内,逼迫阳气浮越于外,临床表现为面红、烦热、口渴、脉大等假热之象。

12. *Yin* collapse or *yang* collapse refers to a critical morbid state due to sudden and excessive loss of *yin* fluid or *yang qi*. 本句中的 yin collapse or *yang* collapse 指的是阴阳亡失。

Task One   Reading Comprehension

1. Which of the following is **NOT** mentioned as the result of the fight between pathogenic factors and the healthy *qi* of the body?

   A. Exuberance and decline of healthy *qi* and pathogenic factors

   B. Disharmony between *qi* and body fluid

   C. Disharmony between *yin* and *yang*

   D. Dysfunction of the viscera and meridians

2. What is the cause of a deficiency syndrome?

   A. Insufficiency of healthy *qi*

   B. Weak constitution

   C. Superabundance of pathogenic factors

   D. Disharmony between *yin* and *yang*

3. Which of the following is **NOT** the cause of relative debilitation of *yang*?

   A. Congenital deficiency

   B. Consumption of *yang qi* due to prolonged illness

   C. Postnatal malnutrition and endogenous impairment due to overstrain

   D. Loss of essence

4. Which of the following is the most serious condition?

   A. Mutual consumption between *yin* and *yang*

   B. *Yin-yang* repulsion

   C. *Yin* collapse or *yang* collapse

   D. Disharmony between *yin* and *yang*

5. What does repulsion mean?

   A. refusal   B. reply   C. decline   D. noun form of "repel"

Task Two   Vocabulary

1. Directions: Complete the following phrases respectively according to its corresponding meaning or equivalent in Chinese within the brackets.

1) _____ (发展) and changes of disease

2) Physical _____ (困乏)

3) relative _____ (平衡) between *yin* and *yang*

4) _____ (功能失调) of the viscera and meridians

5) _____ (先天的) deficiency

6) spiritual and physical _____ (疲乏)

7) lusterless _____ (面色)

8) _____ of breath (气促)

9) feverish sensation over _____ (五心)

10) _____ (盛) of pathogenic factors

11) _____ (畏惧) of cold

12) bone _____ (蒸)

13) true cold with _____ (假热)

14) exuberance *yang* _____ (排斥) *yin*

15) *yang* _____ (亡阳)

16) _____ (催吐的) therapy

17) *yin* _____ (损害) affecting *yang*

18) _____ (潮热)

19) loss of _____ (精气夺)

20) _____ (盗汗)

2. Fill in the blanks with the words from the box and change the form when necessary.

lusterless	deficiency	hypofunction	sole	congenital
mechanism	occurrence	equilibrium	malnutrition	pathogenesis
scanty	dysphoric	coarse	indigestion	disharmony

1) There are widespread shortages of food and the levels of severe acute _____ are still high, especially among children.

2) What's a physical _____ that could lead to differences between these two cells at this very early stage of development?

3) The greater one's inner _____ , the keener the need to create a harmonious life.

4) Renal _____ is not only a sign of mortality of cardiovascular disease, but also one pathogenic factor among them.

5) The exact _____ of this disease is still unknown.

6) The greatest _____ of coronary heart disease is in those over 65.

7) Her _____ hurts after a long day of walking.

8) I paused in the hall to take three deep breaths to restore my _____.

9) When John was 17, he died of _____ heart disease.

10) Now if we have _____, it's very difficult to enjoy food.

11) The cold, pale sunlight fell on their gloomy faces, long hair and _____ eyes.

12) Objective：To establish the mouse model of _____ of both *qi* and blood.

13) Mining firms claim some success in influencing their workers' nocturnal habits, though hard evidence of changed behavior is _____.

14) Some people have a _____ fascination with crime.

15) Now, the Food and Drug Administration has approved the drug for treating premenstrual _____ disorder, a serious form of premenstrual syndrome.

Task Three　Writing

Please rewrite the text in a form of abstract (about 150 words).

Terminology

Basic Terminology of Etiology and pathogenesis

Terminology	WHO	WFCMS
六淫	six excesses	six excesses
三因学说	无	theory of three types of disease cause
怒伤肝	无	anger damaging liver
喜伤心	无	over-joy damaging heart
思伤脾	无	though damaging spleen
忧伤肺	无	anxiety damaging lung
恐伤肾	无	fear damaging kidney
怒则气上	无	rage causing *qi* rising
喜则气缓	无	over-joy causing *qi* to slacken
悲则气消	无	sorrow causing *qi* consumption
恐则气下	无	fear causing *qi* sinking
惊则气乱	无	fright causing disorder of *qi*
虚证	deficiency pattern/syndrome	deficiency syndrome/pattern
实证	excess pattern/syndrome	excess syndrome/pattern
表证	exterior pattern/syndrome	exterior syndrome/pattern
里证	interior pattern/syndrome	interior syndrome/pattern

continued

Terminology	WHO	WFCMS
正邪相争	struggle between the healthy *qi* and pathogenic *qi*	struggle between healthy *qi* and pathogenic *qi*
邪气盛则实,精气夺则虚	无	exuberance of pathogen causing excess syndrome, lack of essential *qi* causing deficiency syndrome
阴阳格拒	*yin-yang* repulsion	无
真寒假热	true cold with false heat	true cold with false heat
真热假寒	true heat with false cold	true heat with false cold
阳盛格阴	exuberant *yang* repelling *yin*	exuberant *yang* repelling *yin*
阴盛格阳	exuberant *yin* repelling *yang*	exuberant *yin* repelling *yang*
亡阴	*yin* collapse	*yin* exhaustion
亡阳	*yang* collapse	*yang* exhaustion

本书配套数字教学资源

微信扫描二维码，加入中医英语读者交流圈，获取配套教学视频、学习课件、课后习题和沟通交流平台等板块内容，夯实基础知识

Tell me about the information collected from inquiry, observation and palpation so as to enable me to experience it myself and have a full understanding of it.

令言而可知，视而可见，扪而可得，令验于己而发蒙解惑①。

Unit 6   The Four Diagnostic Methods

Warming-up

Before You Listen (Watch)

In this section you will hear a short passage about "Four Diagnosis". The following words and phrases may be of help.

stereotypical /ˌsterɪə'tɪpɪkl/	a.	常规的，模式化的
reflux /'riːflʌks/	n.	逆流
urination /ˌjʊərɪ'neɪʃn/	n.	排尿
bowel /'baʊəl/	n.	肠

While You Listen (Watch)

Listen to the passage carefully and fill in each of the blanks marked from 1) to 10) according to what you have heard.

So these are all key questions to be used to 1) _____ very important diagnostic criteria in regard to how Chinese medicine diagnoses illnesses at this ease.

The last skill here "qie" is 2) _____. So the most famous "qie" is pulse 3) _____ and literally channel palpation. So in the pulse diagnosis, the physician is actually feeling three areas of the 4) _____ artery and feeling not only the 5) _____, the 6) _____, and the 7) _____ of pulse, but also feeling each individual position. The first position is known as the "cun", the second is the "guan", and the third is the "chi". And each of these actually also 8) _____ to certain organs in the person's body.

_____

① 《素问·举痛论篇》，李照国译。

So at the end of this large intake, the questioning, the listening, the smelling, the asking, the palpating we were given all of these 9) _____ data, and we have to put these into a concrete diagnosis all together, and then we do our pattern 10) _____ and differential diagnosis as well.

After You Listen(Watch)

Please discuss with your partner the following questions and give your presentation to the class.

1) What does complexion observation imply?

2) What aspects should a doctor inquiry about when diagnosing disease?

3) What are the three positions for a doctor to take a patient's pulse? Can you explain the reason?

4) What are the advantages of the four diagnostic methods in TCM?

Reading

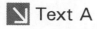 Text A

BEFORE CLASS

1. Quest for Definition

Directions: Explore online the definitions of the following terms from Text A and prepare a unique one-minute oral presentation for your class.

1) pulse-taking method

2) loss of spirit

3) deficiency heat

4) chief complaint

5) exuberance of *yang*

6) blood stasis

2. Text-based Activities

Directions: Read carefully the part of Text A that corresponds to your task, and then prepare a unique one-minute oral presentation for your class.

PERFORMANCE IN CLASS

Your Task

1) What is your understanding of the four diagnostic methods in TCM?

2) What aspects does the inspection method cover?

3) What does the history of present illness include?

4) What kind of syndromes do different complexions indicate?

5) Why does the pulse-taking method choose *cunkou* as the part to diagnose disease?

The Four Diagnostic Methods in TCM

1   The four diagnostic methods in traditional Chinese medicine (TCM) include inspection, listening and smelling, inquiry as well as pulse-taking and **palpation**. Since the human body is an organic whole, local pathological changes may affect the whole body and can be detected from the manifestations of the sensory organs, limbs and surface of the body. "Inspection of the exterior manifestations will enable one to understand the interior conditions; diagnosis of the exterior manifestations will enable one to know the interior states. This is due to the fact that the functions of the internal organs often have their external manifestations①." This quotation from *Dan Xi Xin Fa*② (*Zhu Danxi's Experience in Practicing Medicine*) is a convincing explanation for the application of the four diagnostic methods in TCM.

2   Inspection means that the doctor purposefully observes the whole body or local regions and **excreta** of the patient in order to understand the pathological conditions. The inspection covers such aspects as the vitality, spirit, complexion, posture, physical build and movement.

3   Spirit is the demonstration of life activities. That is why the *Su Wen* (*Plain Conversation*) states that "Loss of spirit causes death while maintenance of spirit ensures life③." The manifestations of spirit vary, but the inspection of spirit mainly concentrates on the states of the eyes, facial expressions and movement of the body. The maintenance of spirit indicates sufficiency of essence and *qi*. Loss of spirit is the sign indicating exhaustion of essence, *qi* and vitality. The manifestations of loss of spirit include unconsciousness, incoherent speech, **carphology**, blurred vision, dull ocular expressions, grayish complexion, indifferent facial expressions, slow reactions, abnormal **respiration**, extreme emaciation, etc. False condition of spirit refers to sudden spurt of vitality prior to collapse. Insufficiency of spirit refers to mild loss of vitality usually seen in patients with deficiency syndrome, the manifestations of which are dispiritedness, **amnesia**, **somnolence**, low voice and no desire to speak, lassitude and slow movement, etc. Abnormal changes of spirit include restlessness, **delirium** and coma, mania and **epilepsy**, etc.

4   Inspection of complexion means observing the facial changes in color and luster. Generally speaking, reddish complexion indicates heat syndromes; whitish complexion indicates cold and deficiency syndrome; yellowish complexion indicates deficiency and dampness syndromes; bluish

---

①   Inspection of the exterior manifestations will enable one to understand the interior conditions; diagnosis of the exterior manifestations will enable one to know the interior states. This is due to the fact that the functions of the internal organs often have their external manifestations：欲知其内者，当以观乎外；诊于外者，斯以知其内。盖有诸内者，必形诸外。

②   *Dan Xi Xin Fa* (*Zhu Danxi's Experience in Practicing Medicine*)：朱震亨的《丹溪心法》。

③   Loss of spirit causes death while maintenance of spirit ensures life：得神者昌，失神者亡。

complexion suggests pain and cold syndrome, blood stasis and convulsion; and blackish complexion shows deficiency of the kidney, blood stasis and fluid retention.

5   Inspection of posture, physical build and movement covers various aspects, such as physical conditions, physical activities, sensory organs, nine orifices, skin, finger veins, secreta, excreta, tongue and coating. Among them, inspection of the tongue is most frequently used in TCM to diagnose disease which is based on four main items: the tongue body color, indicating the conditions of blood, nutrient *qi* and *yin* organs; the tongue body shape, indicating the state of blood and nutrient *qi* and reflecting conditions of fullness or deficiency; the coating, indicating the state of the *yang* organs and reflecting conditions of heat, cold, fullness and deficiency; the moisture, indicating the state of the body fluids.

6   The diagnostic method of listening and smelling is to listen to the voice of speaking, respiration, coughing, vomiting, hiccup, belching, sighing, sneezing and borborygmus, and also to smell the odors emitted from the patient as well as the secreta and excreta. Take voice and breath for example. Under pathological conditions, low and weak voice indicates deficiency syndrome; sonorous voice suggests excess syndrome; rough and asthmatic breath indicates exogenous excess syndrome; weak and short breath suggests deficiency syndrome due to internal injury. Take smell for another example. Sour and foul smell in the mouth indicates retention of food in the stomach; putrid and foul smell in the mouth suggests gingivitis or internal ulcer; foul sweating is usually caused by interior exuberance of heat-toxin; sour and foul feces indicates stagnation in the stomach and intestines; stinking and loose stool suggests cold in the stomach and intestine.

7   Inquiry is a diagnostic method to understand the occurrence and progression of disease, previous treatment, present subjective symptoms and other things concerning the disease by asking the patient or his or her companion. The content of inquiry includes the chief complaints, history of present illness, anamnesis, personal history and family history. The history of present illness includes the onset of disease and present symptoms such as cold, heat, sweat, pain, discomfort, diet, appetite, sleep, urination, defecation, menstruation and leukorrhagia. For female patients, the gynecological matters should also be inquired. For example, menorrhagia may indicate heat in the blood or *qi* deficiency; hypomenorrhea may suggest blood deficiency and stagnation due to cold pathological factor or dysfunction of the thoroughfare vessel (TV) and conception vessel (CV)①. To inquire about anamnesis is helpful for syndrome differentiation and clinical administration of medicine. Since some diseases are infectious and hereditary, the inquiry of family history should not be neglected.

8   Pulse-taking and palpation are the diagnostic methods performed by pressing certain parts of the body to examine the patients. The former is done on the radial artery posterior to the wrist to examine the conditions of the pulse. The latter is done by touching and pressing the skin and muscle, hand and foot as well as chest and abdomen for the purpose of detecting the pathological

---

①   thoroughfare vessel (TV) and conception vessel (CV)：冲脉和任脉,《灵枢·五音五味》记载:"冲脉、任脉皆起于胞中。"

changes.

9   Pulse-taking is the most frequently used method in TCM to diagnose disease. Since blood circulates in the vessels all through the body, the pathological changes in the whole body can be detected from the vessels. In TCM, the part that is selected for taking pulse is the superficial part of the radial artery posterior to the wrist known as *cunkou*. Early morning is the best time to take the pulse for the body being in its calmest state at that time. Usually the physician takes the pulse and makes distinctions of its depth, speed, width, strength, rhythm, length, overall shape and quality.

10   The following are some of the commonly encountered pulse conditions and their significance:

Floating pulse (fu mai): Exterior syndrome (floating and forceful pulse indicating exterior excess syndrome① while floating and weak pulse indicating exterior deficiency syndrome②);

Sunken pulse (chen mai): Interior syndrome (deep and forceful pulse indicating interior excess syndrome while sunken and weak pulse indicating interior deficiency syndrome);

Slow pulse (chi mai): Cold syndrome (slow and forceful pulse indicating excess-cold syndrome③ while slow and weak pulse indicating deficiency-cold syndrome④);

Rapid pulse (shuo mai): Heat syndrome (rapid and forceful pulse indicating excess-heat while rapid and weak pulse indicating deficiency heat);

Weak pulse (xu mai): Deficiency syndrome (often deficiency of both *qi* and blood);

Excess pulse (shi mai): Excess syndrome;

Slippery pulse (hua mai): Retention of phlegm and food, excess heat;

Unsmooth pulse (se mai): Consumption of essence, deficiency of blood, stagnation of *qi* and stasis of blood;

Surging pulse (hong mai): Exuberance of heat and pathogenic factors;

Thin pulse (xi mai): Deficiency of *yin* blood and dampness;

Soggy pulse (ru mai): Various conditions of deficiency and dampness;

Wiry pulse (xian mai): Liver and gallbladder disease, various kinds of pain problems, phlegm and retention of fluid;

Tight pulse (jin mai): Pain and cold;

Rapid irregular **intermittent** pulse (cu mai): Excess-heat due to *yang* exuberance⑤, phlegm, retention of fluid and food;

Knotted pulse (jie mai): *Qi* stagnation due to *yin* predomination⑥, phlegm stagnation and blood stasis;

Intermittent pulse (dai mai): Declination of visceral *qi*, wind and pain syndrome, fright and

---

①   exterior excess syndrome: 表实证。
②   exterior deficiency syndrome: 表虚证。
③   excess-cold syndrome: 实寒证。
④   deficiency-cold syndrome: 虚寒证。
⑤   *yang* exuberance: 阳盛。
⑥   *yin* predomination: 阴胜。

traumatic injury. (1,236 words)

New Words and Expressions

palpation /pæl'peɪʃn/ *n*. examination by touching (诊断时)摸;触

excreta /ɪk'skriːtə/ *n*. substance that is excreted 排泄物

carphology /kɑː'fɒlədʒɪ/ *n*. an aimless semiconscious plucking at the bedclothes observed in conditions of exhaustion or stupor or in high fevers 摸空,捉空摸床(抓摸想象中的物品或抓扯床单的行为,是精神错乱者的典型症状)

respiration /respɪ'reɪʃ(ə)n/ *n*. the movement of air or dissolved gases into and out of the lungs 呼吸

amnesia /æm'niːzɪə/ *n*. loss of memory due usually to brain injury, shock, fatigue, repression, or illness 遗忘症,善忘,健忘

somnolence /'sɒmnələns/ *n*. the quality or state of being drowsy, sleepiness 嗜睡,瞌睡

delirium /dɪ'lɪrɪəm/ *n*. an acute mental disturbance characterized by confused thinking and disrupted attention usually accompanied by disordered speech and hallucinations 精神错乱,说胡话

epilepsy /'epɪlepsɪ/ *n*. any of various disorders marked by abnormal electrical discharges in the brain and typically manifested by sudden brief episodes of altered or diminished consciousness, involuntary movements, or convulsions 癫痫,羊痫风

convulsion /kən'vʌlʃ(ə)n/ *n*. an abnormal violent and involuntary contraction or series of contractions of the muscles 惊厥,震动

retention /rɪ'tenʃ(ə)n/ *n*. abnormal retaining of a fluid or secretion in a body cavity 保留,滞留

secreta /sɪ'kriːtə/ *n*. substances secreted by a cell, tissue, or organ; the products of secretion(细胞、组织或器官的)分泌物

hiccup /'hɪkʌp/ *n*. sudden involuntary stopping of the breath with a sharp gulp-like sound, often recurring at short intervals 打嗝,呃逆

belching /beltʃɪŋ/ *n*. sending out gas from the stomach noisily through the mouth 打嗝

borborygmus /ˌbɔːbə'rɪgməs/ *n*. gurgling sound in the intestines 肠鸣

sonorous /'sɒnərəs/ *a*. having a pleasant full deep sound 雄浑的;浑厚的

asthmatic /æs'mætɪk/ *a*. relating to or suffering from asthma 气喘的;似患气喘的

putrid /'pjuːtrɪd/ *a*. (rotting and therefore) foul-smelling; noxious (因腐烂)发臭的;有害的

gingivitis /ˌdʒɪndʒɪ'vaɪtɪs/ *n*. inflammation of the gums 齿龈炎

stink /stɪŋk/ *v*. have a very unpleasant and offensive smell 有臭味;发臭

anamnesis /ænəm'niːsɪs/ *n*. memory; previous medical record 记忆力;既往病历

defecation /ˌdefə'keɪʃn/ *n*. the elimination of fecal waste through the anus 排便;澄清,净化

leukorrhagia /ljuːkəu'reɪdʒɪə/ *n*. vaginal discharge of whitish liquid substance 白带过多

gynecological /ˌgaɪnɪkə'lɒdʒɪkəl/ *a*. of or relating to or practicing gynecology 妇科的;妇产科医学的

menorrhagia /menə'reɪdʒɪə/ *n*. abnormally heavy or prolonged menstruation [妇产] 月经过多

hypomenorrhea /haɪpə,menə'rɪəː/ *n*. extremely light menstrual blood flow [妇产] 月经过少

administration /ədˌmɪnɪ'streɪʃn/ *n*. (medicines or drugs) usage (药的)服法、用法、给药

radial /ˈreɪdɪəl/ *a.* of radius 桡骨的

intermittent /ˌɪntəˈmɪtənt/ *a.* continually stopping and then starting again；not constant 间歇的

traumatic /trɔːˈmætɪk/ *a.* of or relating to a physical injury or wound to the body(心理)创伤的，(生理)外伤的

FOLLOW-UP ACTIVITIES

Task One　Comprehension Check

1. Questions for Discussion

1）How do we justify the application of the four diagnostic methods in TCM?

2）What is the difference between loss of spirit and insufficiency of spirit?

3）Why is the inquiry about anamnesis important when doctors diagnose diseases?

4）What are the characteristics of a normal pulse?

2. Chart Completion

INTRODUCTION：(para. 1)

　　The four diagnostic methods in traditional Chinese medicine (TCM) include 1)_____ _____ , listening and smelling, inquiry as well as pulse-taking and 2)_____ _____ . Diagnosis of the exterior 3)_____ will enable one to know the interior states.

INSPECTION METHOD：(para. 2 – 5)

- Inspection of spirit mainly concentrates on the states of the eyes, facial expressions and 4)_____ of the body.
- Inspection of 5)_____ means observing the facial changes in color and luster.
- Inspection of posture, physical build and movement covers various aspects, such as physical conditions, physical activities, sensory organs, nine 6)_____ , skin, finger veins, secreta, excreta, tongue and 7)_____ .

LISTENING AND SMELLING METHOD：(para. 6)

　　The diagnostic method of listening and smelling is to listen to the voice of speaking, 8)_____ , coughing, vomiting, hiccup, belching, sighing, sneezing and borborygmus, and to smell the odors emitted from the patient as well as the 9)_____ _____ and excreta.

INQUIRY METHOD：(para. 7)

　　Inquiry is a diagnostic method to understand the 10)_____ and progress of disease, previous treatment, present 11)_____ symptoms and other things concerning the disease by asking the patient or his or her 12)_____ _____ .

PULSE-TAKING AND PALPATION METHOD：（para. 8－10）
　　Pulse-taking is done on the radial artery 13) ＿＿＿＿＿＿＿＿＿＿＿ to the wrist to examine the conditions of the pulse and palpation is done by touching and pressing the skin and muscle, hand and foot as well as chest and abdomen for the purpose of detecting the 14)＿＿＿＿＿＿＿＿＿＿ changes. In TCM, the part that is selected for taking pulse is the 15) ＿＿＿＿＿＿＿＿＿＿＿ part of the radial artery posterior to the wrist known as *cunkou*.

Task Two　Vocabulary

1. Directions：Complete the following phrases respectively according to its corresponding meaning or equivalent in Chinese within the brackets.

1) ＿＿＿＿＿＿＿（有机的）whole
2) ＿＿＿＿＿＿＿＿＿（病理的）change
3) ＿＿＿＿＿＿＿＿（感官的）organs
4) external ＿＿＿＿＿＿＿＿＿（表现）
5) local ＿＿＿＿＿＿＿＿＿（部位）
6) ＿＿＿＿＿＿＿＿＿（维持）of spirit
7) ＿＿＿＿＿＿＿（面部的）expression
8) ＿＿＿＿＿＿＿＿＿（充足）of essence
9) ＿＿＿＿＿＿＿（耗竭）of essence
10) ＿＿＿＿＿＿＿＿＿（语无伦次的）speech
11) ＿＿＿＿＿＿＿＿＿（模糊的）vision
12) ＿＿＿＿＿＿＿＿＿（异常的）respiration
13) ＿＿＿＿＿＿＿＿＿（极端的）emaciation
14) ＿＿＿＿＿＿＿＿＿（喷出）of vitality
15) ＿＿＿＿＿＿（有说服力的）explanation
16) color and ＿＿＿＿＿＿＿＿＿（光泽）
17) ＿＿＿＿＿＿＿＿＿（水液）retention
18) finger ＿＿＿＿＿＿＿＿＿（静脉）
19) ＿＿＿＿＿＿＿＿＿（营养的）*qi*
20) ＿＿＿＿＿＿＿＿＿（实）syndrome
21) ＿＿＿＿＿＿＿＿＿（难闻的）smell
22) ＿＿＿＿＿＿＿＿＿（盛）of heat-toxin
23) ＿＿＿＿＿＿＿＿＿（发作）of disease
24) ＿＿＿＿＿＿＿＿＿（浑厚的）voice
25) clinical ＿＿＿＿＿＿＿（用药,给药）
26) infectious and ＿＿＿＿＿＿（遗传的）
27) radial ＿＿＿＿＿＿＿＿＿（动脉）
28) ＿＿＿＿＿＿＿＿＿（漂浮的）pulse
29) ＿＿＿＿＿＿＿（创伤的）injury
30) ＿＿＿＿＿＿＿＿＿（打结的）pulse

2. Match the following words with their proper meanings.

Column I	Column II
1) vitality	a. the natural color and condition of the skin on a person's face
2) complexion	b. energy and enthusiasm
3) ocular	c. extreme leanness (usually caused by starvation or disease)
4) indifferent	d. having or showing no interest in sb./sth.
5) emaciation	e. connected with the eyes
6) lassitude	f. a thin layer covering something
7) mania	g. to throw or give off or out

continued

Column I	Column II
8) coating	h. a state of feeling very tired in mind or body; lack of energy
9) respiration	i. the movement of air or dissolved gases into and out of the lungs
10) deficiency	j. the quality or state of being exuberant
11) emit	k. a mood disorder
12) exuberance	l. lack of an adequate quantity or number
13) hereditary	m. the state of being predominant over others
14) surge	n. given to a child by its parents before it is born
15) predomination	o. to move quickly and with force in a particular direction

3. Fill in the blanks with the words from the box and change the form when necessary.

vitality	complexion	ocular	indifferent	emaciation
lassitude	retention	coating	respiration	sneeze
emit	palpation	hereditary	surge	predominance

1) And the diversity that refugees (难民) bring is welcomed, adding _____ and variety to the state's arts and cultural scene.

2) Her cheeks were sunken, _____ sallow (蜡黄的), her tiny frame emaciated and frail.

3) Between 2016 and 2018, pollution of fine particulate matter (细颗粒物) — tiny particles that are _____ whenever we burn anything — rose by more than 5 percent.

4) A sudden feeling of _____, of intense weariness, spread over Vera's limbs

5) Their current study is examining whether levels of brain synchrony during class predict _____ of material learned.

6) Under the _____ of dust and cobwebs, he discovered a fine French Louis XVI clock.

7) For the last decade, the role of the microbiome (微生物) in _____ health was controversial.

8) Modern CT scans, for example, perform better than even the best surgeons' _____ of a painful abdomen in detecting appendicitis.

9) In 1994, the physician founded Sickle Cell Foundation Nigeria, with a mission to provide support for people with sickle-cell (镰状红细胞) disease — a _____ blood disorder that affects 20 million individuals worldwide.

10) Once reserved for China's elites, ejiao (阿胶) is now marketed to the country's booming middle class, causing demand to _____.

11) So that means kicking our metabolism (新陈代谢) into high gear, increasing our _____, our heart rate increases.

12) When I look at my career at midlife, I realize that in many ways I've become the kind of doctor I never thought I'd be: often impatient, at times _____ or paternalistic(家长式作

风的）.

13) This male _____ is, of course, due to prenatal ultrasound（产前超声波检查）, parental preference and sex-selective abortion（堕胎）.

14) The infection is highly contagious（传染性的）, spreading easily when a person coughs or _____ .

15) The fatal disease attacks deer's brains, leading to _____ and abnormal behavior.

Task Three   Translation

1. Translate the following medical expressions into English

1) 神色形态
2) 精神活动
3) 精充气足
4) 表情淡漠
5) 主色与客色
6) 四肢抽搐
7) 湿热动风
8) 邪毒内陷
9) 肌肤甲错
10) 饥不欲食
11) 四诊合参
12) 面部表情
13) 预后良好
14) 精神不振
15) 五色主病
16) 口眼歪斜
17) 虚火上炎
18) 大肠热结
19) 光剥舌
20) 脉象

2. Translate the following sentences into Chinese or English

1) Inspection is a diagnostic method of observing general or local changes of spirit, complexion and physical conditions.

2) Inquiry is a diagnostic method used to understand the occurrence, development, present subjective symptoms and other things concerning the diseases by asking the patients or their companions.

3) Local pathological changes may involve the whole body and the viscera, which can be manifested in various aspects.

4) Bluish color indicates cold syndrome, pain syndrome, blood stasis and infantile convulsion.

5) Pulse-taking and palpitation refer to the diagnostic method of feeling the pulse and palpating the stomach and abdomen, foot and hand as well as other regions of the patients.

6) 在临床应用中,只有四诊合参才能得到正确的诊断。(enable ... to)

7) 黄色舌苔一般主里证、热证,由热邪熏灼所致。(due to)

8) 切脉是通过按压手腕后面的桡骨动脉来探知脉的情况。(posterior to)

9) 辨证是基于望、闻、问、切四诊法收集的症状和身体指标来诊断疾病的过程。(based on)

10) 常色指人在正常生理状态下的面部色泽。(under ... condition)

3. Translate the following passage into English

　　中医诊断主要由医生自主通过望、闻、问、切等方法收集患者资料,不依赖于各种复杂的仪器设备。中医干预既有药物,也有针灸、推拿、拔罐、刮痧等非药物疗法。许多非药物疗法不需要复杂器具,其所需器具(如小夹板、刮痧板、火罐等)往往可以就地取材,易于推广使用。

◥ Text B

Pulse Diagnosis

1　Inspection, listening and smelling, inquiry and pulse taking and palpation are the four examinations of traditional Chinese medicine（TCM）, among which pulse taking is the most mysterious and extremely **subjective** form of diagnosis. Pulse diagnosis is important. On the one hand, it can give very detailed information on the state of the internal organs, and on the other hand, it reflects the whole complex of *qi* and blood. The pulse can be seen as a clinical manifestation, a sign like any other such as thirst, **insomnia** or a red face.

2　Traditionally, the best time for taking the pulse is in the early morning when the *yin* is calm and the *yang* has not yet come forth. It is important for the practitioner to regulate and balance his or her own breathing pattern in order to be better **attuned** to the patient's *qi* and to become more receptive. One inspiration and one **expiration** make up one cycle of respiration, and the normal ratio is four to five beats to one respiration. The patient's arm should be **horizontal** and should not be held higher than the level of the heart. The examination is made upon both the right and left wrists with three fingers. The middle finger is first laid on the head of the **radius**, then followed by the index and ring fingers. The thumb rests upon the dorsum of the **carpus**.

3　The pulse is divided into three parts known as *cun*, *guan* and *chi*, with index finger, middle finger and ring finger pressing on these respective areas. The indications of them are very important, each variety or combination of varieties revealing a distinct disease. Thus a superficial pulse, which belongs to *yang*, points to complaints externally due to the six pathogenic factors — wind, cold, summer-heat, dampness, dryness and fire. If a pulse is superficial and rapid, it indicates wind and heat; if it is superficial and weak, it shows blood deficiency. If it is superficial and tight, it signifies wind and cold; if it is replete, it indicates **rheumatism**. A combination of superficial and soft pulses denotes

subjective /səbˈdʒektɪv/ *adj.* 主观的

insomnia /ɪnˈsɒmnɪə/ *n.* 失眠

attune /əˈtjuːn/ *v.* 使协调

expiration /ˌekspɪˈreɪʃn/ *n.* 呼气

horizontal /ˌhɒrɪˈzɒntəl/ *adj.* 水平的

radius /ˈreɪdɪəs/ *n.* 桡骨
carpus /ˈkɑːpəs/ *n.* 手腕;腕骨

rheumatism /ˈruːməˌtɪzəm/ *n.* 风湿,风湿病

sunstroke; superficial and hollow, **hemorrhage**; superficial and thre_dy, fatigue due to overwork; superficial and faint, seminal weakness; superficial and scattered, exhaustion and collapse; superficial and wiry, **indigestion**; and superficial and slippery, wind and phlegm. A deep pulse, which belongs to *yin*, indicates disease due to internal impairment. If the pulse is deep and slow, it shows weakness and cold; if the pulse is deep and rapid, it signifies **latent** heat; if the pulse is tight, it means **colic** due to chills; if the pulse is slow, it indicates accumulation of water. A deep and slippery pulse points to indigestion; while a deep and hidden pulse indicates vomiting and diarrhea.

4   The above is a brief analysis of the various types of pulse and their significance in diagnostics. TCM doctors mainly depend on the examination of the pulse to diagnose disease and believe that analysis of the pulse can predict the result of an illness. For instance, in wasting diseases, the pulse is usually weak and quick; if it is thin and small, death is certain. In cases of loss of blood, the **prognosis** is favorable if the pulse is hollow, small and slow; but if it is strong, large and quick, it is unfavorable.

5   In the theory of pulse there are some special pulses that indicate **impending** death. If the pulse resembles the pecking of a bird, water dripping from a roof crack, death may be expected within four days. If the pulse resembles feathers blown by the wind, or feathers brushing against the skin, it indicates serious disease of the lungs and death will be due within three days. It is a sign of fatal kidney trouble and death may happen within four days if the pulse is like the snapping of a cord or like the flipping of the finger against stone. When the liver ceases to perform its functions, the pulse is felt like the **string** of a new bow or like touching the edge of a sword. In this case the patient will die within eight days. If the pulse resembles the rapid rolling of peas, death may be expected in one day. A pulse felt like a fish or shrimp darting about in the water or like water **oozing** from a spring, it is a fatal symptom.

6   An important point, which should also be taken into consideration, when taking a pulse, is the normal variation due to season, constitution, age and gender. In spring the pulse is taut and tremulous like a musical string; in summer it is full and overflowing; in autumn it is **elastic**; and in winter it is deep like a

hemorrhage /'hemərɪdʒ/ *n.* 出血

indigestion /ˌɪndɪ'dʒestʃən/ *n.* 消化不良

latent /'leɪtənt/ *adj.* 潜在的
colic /'kɔlɪk/ *n.* 疝气；腹绞痛

prognosis /prɔg'nəusɪs/ *n.* 预后

impending /ɪm'pendɪŋ/ *adj.* 将发生的

string /strɪŋ/ *n.* 弦

ooze /uːz/ *v.* 渗出，泄漏

elastic /ɪ'læstɪk/ *adj.* 有弹性的

stone thrown into water.

7   A thin person's pulse is generally superficial and quick, a heavy person's pulse is usually deep and full. Five beats to one cycle of respiration are normal in a hot-tempered person, but four beats to one cycle of respiration in a person of slow temperament. In elderly patients, the pulse is mostly empty; in young patients, it is large; and in infants it is rapid, about eight beats to one cycle of respiration. Geographically, Northerners often have strong and full pulses, while Southerners have soft and weak pulses.

temperament /ˈtempərəmənt/ n. 性情

8   Differentiation is also made between the pulses of different genders. In man the pulse on the left hand should be large to correspond to *yang*, but in women it should be the opposite because *yin* dominates on the right. Again the *chi* pulse in man is always slow, weak and compressible while in woman it is usually strong, large and long. The examination of pulse sometimes even can tell whether or not a woman is pregnant, or even predict the sex and development of fetus. For instance, in a case of cessation of menstruation with no apparent disease, if the three pulses are slippery, it indicates pregnancy. If they are rapid and scattered, it indicates the patient is three months pregnant.

dominate /ˈdɒmɪneɪt/ v. 支配

9   This is a general summary of the pulse according to doctors of traditional Chinese medicine. To doctors in modern medicine, maybe it is difficult to understand and accept. Perhaps modern doctors, with so many instruments to aid them in diagnosis, have lost many of their faculties of observation, especially the sense of touch. Constant use and pure concentration may have enabled doctors in TCM to develop this power to such an extent that they can tell many things imperceptible to the untrained person. (1,073 words)

faculty /ˈfækəltɪ/ n. 官能

imperceptible /ˌɪmpəˈseptəbl/ adj. 难以察觉的

Notes：

1. when the *yin* is calm and the *yang* has not yet come forth. 阴气未动,阳气未散。
2. the normal ratio is four to five beats to one respiration. 一息四到五至。
3. The pulse is divided into three parts known as cun, guan and chi. 脉分为三个部分,即寸、关、尺。
4. Thus a superficial pulse, which belongs to *yang*, points to complaints externally due to the six pathogenic factors — wind, cold, summer-heat, dampness, dryness and fire. 浮脉属阳,主六淫(风、寒、暑、湿、燥、火)所致之外感疾病。
5. If the pulse resembles the pecking of a bird, water dripping from a roof crack, death may be expected within four days. 脉如雀喙啄食或屋漏残滴,四日死。

6. If the pulse resembles feathers blown by the wind, or feathers brushing against the skin, it indicates serious disease of the lungs and death will be due within three days. 脉如风吹毛,如以毛羽中人肤,乃肺之危重证候,三日死。

7. A pulse felt like a fish or shrimp darting about in the water or like water oozing from a spring, it is a fatal symptom. 脉如鱼翔或虾游或水从泉渗,属危候。

8. In spring the pulse is taut and tremulous like a musical string; in summer it is full and overflowing; in autumn it is elastic; and in winter it is deep like a stone thrown into water. 脉象春弦、夏洪、秋浮、冬沉。

9. In man the pulse on the left hand should be large to correspond to *yang*, but in women it should be the opposite because *yin* dominates on the right. 男子左手脉大,阳脉常盛;妇人右手脉大,阴脉常盛。

10. Again the *chi* pulse in man is always slow, weak and compressible while in woman it is usually strong, large and long. 男子尺脉恒弱,女子尺脉恒盛。

Task One   Reading Comprehension

1. The best time to take pulse is in the _____ .
   - A. afternoon
   - B. early morning at sunrise
   - C. evening
   - D. either morning or afternoon

2. When a doctor takes pulse, he or she should be _____ .
   - A. cool
   - B. concentrated
   - C. enthusiastic
   - D. both A and B

3. Which pulse points to complaints externally due to the six pathogenic factors?
   - A. Superficial pulse.   B. Slow pulse.   C. Taut pulse.   D. Quick pulse.

4. If a patient's pulse condition feels like the rapid rolling of peas, the death may be within _____ .
   - A. one day   B. two days   C. three days   D. four days

5. A heavy person's pulse is usually _____ .
   - A. deep and slow
   - B. deep and slippery
   - C. deep and full
   - D. deep and taut

Task Two   Vocabulary

1. **Directions: Complete the following phrases respectively according to its corresponding meaning or equivalent in Chinese within the brackets.**

1) pulse taking and _____ (切诊)   2) four _____ (四诊)

3) _____ (详细的) information   4) one cycle of _____ (呼吸)

5) _____ pulse (浮脉)   6) _____ (致病的) factors

7) blood _____ (虚)   8) _____ (细脉) pulse

9) _____ (滑脉) pulse   10) _____ (沉脉) pulse

11) _____（伏的）heat

12) _____（积聚）of water

13) _____（消耗的）diseases

14) favorable _____（预后）

15) _____（即将到来的）death

16) _____（危重的）symptom

17) _____（散脉）pulse

18) _____（暴躁的）person

19) _____（现代）medicine

20) _____（能力）of observation

2. Fill in the blanks with the words from the box and change the form when necessary.

inspect	superficial	horizontal	accumulate	fatigue
diagnose	collapse	complain	fatal	insomnia
elastic	prognosis	impending	temperament	dominate

1) Any _____ vein may become varicosed（脉肿的；曲张的）, which means twisted and enlarged, but they are most commonly found in the legs.

2) The federal government only requires that _____ teams include a registered nurse.

3) Complications may be common; a possible link between coffee drinking and _____ was identified more than 100 years ago.

4) At the emergency room, doctors were given a box of expired masks, and when they tried to put them on, the _____ bands snapped（断裂）.

5) It is essential that physicians communicate openly and honestly with patients on the disease, treatment options and _____ .

6) Everything in nature is vertical（垂直的,向上的）as it tries to reach the sun; if you see something _____ , like a branch on the ground, chances are humans were there.

7) According to this hypothesis, the _____ of beta amyloid（β-淀粉样蛋白）in the brain is the primary cause of the disease.

8) The breathable and comfortable pieces support major muscles during activity to promote blood flow, reduce _____ and help prevent injuries from overuse.

9) Following her _____ , Jane began medication which suppressed the virus and made HIV levels virtually undetectable in her system.

10) Occasionally the hemorrhoid（痔疮）will _____ , and when it does, that hurts.

11) There is nothing like an _____ surgery to get smokers to kick the habit for good.

12) Studies show that parents react sensitively to the innate _____ of their offspring and adapt their upbringing accordingly.

13) Cases predominately involve the toes, sole, rim of the foot and heels, with itching and irritation a common _____ among patients.

14) Two people were reportedly diagnosed with the highly infectious, potentially _____ pneumonic plague in a hospital.

15) Strangely, modern science was long _____ by the idea that to be scientific means to remove consciousness from our explanations, in order to be "objective".

Task Three Writing

Please rewrite the text in a form of abstract（about 150 words）

Terminology

Basic Terminology of TCM Diagnostics

Terminology	WHO	WFCMS
诊法	diagnostic method	diagnostic method
四诊	four examinations	four examinations
望诊	inspection	inspection
望神	inspection of the vitality	inspection of vitality
得神	presence of vitality	presence of vitality
失神	loss of vitality	loss of vitality
少神	lack of vitality	lack of vitality
望色	inspection of the complexion	inspection of complexion
面色	（facial）complexion	complexion
舌诊	tongue diagnosis	tongue inspection
舌象	tongue manifestation	tongue manifestation
舌苔	tongue fur	tongue coating；tongue fur
闻诊	listening and smelling examination	listening and smelling；inquiry
失音	loss of voice	loss of voice
太息	sighing	sighing
问诊	inquiry	无
恶寒	aversion to cold	aversion to cold
畏寒	fear of cold	fear of cold
自汗	spontaneous sweating	spontaneous sweating
盗汗	night sweating	night sweat
脉诊	pulse diagnosis	pulse diagnosis
切诊	palpation	pulse taking and palpation
寸口	wrist pulse	wrist pulse
平脉	normal pulse	normal pulse
病脉	morbid pulse	abnormal pulse
浮脉	floating pulse	floating pulse
沉脉	sunken pulse	deep pulse

continued

Terminology	WHO	WFCMS
迟脉	slow pulse	slow pulse
数脉	rapid pulse	rapid pulse
洪脉	surging pulse	surging pulse
实脉	replete pulse	replete pulse
滑脉	slippery pulse	slippery pulse
弦脉	string-like pulse	wiry pulse
雀啄脉	pecking sparrow pulse	sparrow-pecking pulse
鱼翔脉	waving fish pulse	fish-swimming pulse
虾游脉	darting shrimp pulse	shrimp-darting pulse
屋漏脉	leaking roof pulse	roof-leaking pulse

本书配套数字教学资源

微信扫描二维码，加入中医英语读者交流圈，获取配套教学视频、学习课件、课后习题和沟通交流平台等板块内容，夯实基础知识

It is through the twelve conduit vessels that a person comes to life.

夫十二经脉者，人之所以生①。

Unit 7　The Meridian System

Warming-up

Before you listen（Watch）

In this section you will hear a short passage about "Hand *Tai Yin* Lung Channel"②. The following words and phrases may be of help.

residence /ˈrezɪdəns/	*n.*	住宅，住处；居住	
practitioner /prækˈtɪʃənə(r)/	*n.*	开业者，从业者，执业医生	
wheezing /wiːzɪŋ/	*n.*	喘息	
asthma /ˈæsmə/	*n.*	哮喘，气喘	
thenar /ˈθiːnɑː/	*a.*	鱼际的；拇指球的；手掌的	
eminence /ˈemɪnəns/	*n.*	(骨的表面的)隆起，隆凸，隆突	
congestion /kənˈdʒestʃən/	*n.*	拥挤；拥塞；瘀血	
divergent /daɪˈvɜːdʒənt/	*a.*	分歧的，分叉的	
sinew /ˈsɪnjuː/	*n.*	筋；肌腱	
costal /ˈkɒstl/	*a.*	肋的；肋骨的	

---

① 《灵枢·经别》，Paul U. Unschuld 译。

② "经络"一词现有两种译法：① channel；② meridian。《新牛津英语词典》对两个单词的解释(医学相关)分别为：channel：a tubular passage or duct for liquid(液体的通道或管道)；meridian：(in acupuncture and Chinese medicine) each of a set of pathways in the body along which vital energy is said to flow. (中医针灸)人体精气流经的路径。

目前这两种译法都很流行。"经"译为 channel 取其经络乃气血通行之要道之意；"经"译为 meridian 则反映中医针灸天人合一的理念。世界中医药学会联合会颁布的《中医基本名词术语中英对照国际标准》中"经络"对应英译为 meridian╱channel and collateral；WHO 发布的《针灸经穴名称国际标准化方案》中"经络"对应英译为 meridian and collateral。"经络"现在还有一种较为普遍的译法：当翻译"经络"总体概念时用 meridian，当翻译具体"经(脉)"和"络(脉)"时，分别译成 channel 和 collateral。

While you listen (Watch)

Listen to the passage carefully and fill in each of the blanks marked from 1) to 10) according to what you have heard.

In Chapter 8 of *Su Wen*, it says that the lung holds the office of prime minister and is the 1) _____ of management and 2) _____. It means that the lung is the prime minister to the heart, and the heart is the emperor and 3) _____ over everything, but the lung is the one taking care of day-to-day details. So, there's a strong relationship between the heart and the lung in terms of the governing of the body's functions. And that's why they both sit right next to each other and just sharing a 4) _____ in the upper *jiao*.

We can take a look at the actual pathways of the channel. Here's the 5) _____ Channel. First, the lung channel starts with its internal pathway in the middle *jiao*. Second, the channel connects to the lung and 6) _____. But what we want to pay attention to is if the channel connects to any 7) _____ organs. Actually, the lung channel travels through the stomach organ. This lets us know that we can select points along the lung channel to treat certain stomach conditions like nausea, vomiting, and 8) _____.

Next, we have the 9) _____ Channel. They strengthen the connection between *yin-yang* paired organs. So here we see the divergent channel connecting to the lung and large intestine. Number two, they supply *qi* to the head and face. So again, we see the lung divergent channel going up to the throat leading things like sore throat. And three, divergent channels reconnect to their *yang*-paired primary channel. Here's a summary. We have nasal 10) _____ and throat problems. So those are things that can be treated by points along the lung channel.

After you listen (Watch)

Please discuss with your partner the following questions and give your presentation to the class.

1) According to the lecture, what conditions can be treated by using points on the lung channel?
2) Review what you have learned in the previous units and illustrate the functions and characteristics of the lung.
3) Please introduce the actual pathways of the lung channel in this lecture.
4) Please list the TCM therapies based on the channel / meridian and collateral theory and introduce one of them in detail.
5) According to the Chinese 12 Meridian Clock, the liver channel corresponds to 1 am to 3 am, so what should you do and what will happen to your body if you stay active during this period of time?

Reading

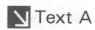 Text A

BEFORE CLASS

1. Quest for Definition

Directions: Explore online the definitions of the following terms from Text A and prepare a unique one-minute oral presentation for your class.

1) twelve regular meridians
2) eight extraordinary meridians
3) fifteen divergent collaterals
4) floating collaterals
5) twelve musculature zones
6) twelve skin divisions

2. Text-based Activities

Directions: Read carefully the part of Text A that corresponds to your task, and then prepare a unique one-minute oral presentation for your class.

PERFORMANCE IN CLASS

Your Task

1) Please summarize the physiological functions of the meridian system in your own words.

2) What are the categories of the meridians?

3) What are the categories of the collaterals?

4) Can you briefly introduce the difference between the three *yin* meridians and the three *yang* meridians of the hand?

5) How can pathogenic factors affect the body through meridians?

Meridian System

1   Meridian system is the most important part of TCM. It serves as the foundation for acupuncture, moxibustion, Tuina and Qigong. The knowledge of human anatomy has played an important role in the development of the theory of meridian system. Its theory focuses on the study of the physiological functions and pathological changes of human body as a whole.

2   The meridian system refers to the pathways for *qi* to circulate in the whole body. These pathways

connect the viscera with the limbs and joints, link the upper part of the body with the lower part and associate the interior portion with the exterior. The meridians are the major trunks of this system while the collaterals are the branches of the system①. Some of the meridian lines are visible on the surface of the body. The meridians run in order and interconnect as a large loop while the collaterals run **reticularly** to **weave** all the viscera, organs, orifices, muscles, skin and bones of the body②.

3   The meridians can be classified into two categories, namely the regular meridians and the extraordinary meridians. There are twelve regular meridians, including three *yin* meridians and three *yang* meridians of the hand and foot③ respectively. They are the main pathways for *qi* to circulate in the body. The twelve regular meridians④ have their starting and ending points inter-connected to form a large loop. There are eight extraordinary meridians⑤, namely the governor vessel, **conception** vessel, **thoroughfare** vessel, belt vessel, *yin* heel vessel⑥, *yang* heel vessel, *yin* link vessel and *yang* link vessel⑦. These extraordinary meridians also link with the twelve regular meridians.

4   The collaterals are the branches of the system. They can be divided into three categories: the divergent collaterals⑧, superficial collaterals⑨ and fine collaterals⑩. The divergent collaterals are the large and major collaterals. Each of the twelve regular meridians has one divergent collateral and so do the governor vessel and conception vessel⑪. Together with the large spleen collateral, there are "fifteen divergent collaterals"⑫. The main function of the divergent branches is to strengthen the connection between every pair of meridians in exterior and interior relation. The superficial collaterals run in the shallow regions of the body and are often visible on the surface of the body. For this reason, they are also called "floating collaterals". The fine collaterals are the smallest and thinnest ones in the body⑬. The twelve **musculature** zones⑭ and twelve skin divisions⑮

---

①   The meridians are the major trunks in this system while the collaterals are the branches of the system：经脉是经络系统的主干，而络脉是经脉的分支。

②   The meridians run in order and interconnect as a large loop while the collaterals run reticularly to weave all the viscera, organs, orifices, muscles, skin and bones of the body：经脉有序运行，并作为一个大循环相互关联，而络脉呈网状运行于人体所有的脏腑、器官、孔窍、肌肉、皮肤和骨骼。

③   three *yin* meridians and three *yang* meridians of the hand and foot：手三阴经、手三阳经、足三阴经、足三阳经。

④   the twelve regular meridians：十二正经，一般指经脉。

⑤   eight extraordinary meridians：奇经八脉。

⑥   *yin* heel vessel：阴蹻脉。

⑦   *yang* link vessel：阳维脉。

⑧   divergent collaterals：别络。

⑨   superficial collaterals：浮络，亦译为"floating collaterals"。

⑩   fine collaterals：孙络。

⑪   Each of the twelve regular meridians has one divergent collateral and so do the governor vessel and conception vessel：十二正经中每条和督脉、任脉都有一条别络。

⑫   Together with the large spleen collateral, there are "fifteen divergent collaterals"：加上脾之大络，总共有"十五别络"。

⑬   The fine collaterals are the smallest and thinnest ones in the body：孙络是人体最细小的络脉。

⑭   twelve musculature zones：十二经筋，经筋具有约束骨骼、屈伸关节、维持人体正常运动功能的作用。

⑮   twelve skin divisions：十二皮部。

are the subsidiary parts of the twelve regular meridians. According to the theory of meridian system, musculature zones form a system through which *qi* from the twelve meridians "retains, accumulates, disperses and connects" in the musculature and joints①. The skin is the region to reflect the functional activities of the twelve regular meridians and the dispersion of the meridian *qi*. That is why the skin of the body is divided into twelve parts, which correspond directly to the twelve meridians.

5　Physiologically, the meridians serve as the pathways for *qi* to circulate in the body. Pathologically, the meridians transmit pathogenic factors into the body. When the meridian *qi* becomes weak or fails to protect the body due to certain factors, exogenous pathogenic factors may invade the body and pathogenic factors will be transmitted into the viscera through the meridian system. Similarly, when the pathological changes have taken place in the viscera, they may be transmitted to the surface of the body through the system of meridians②.

6　Since the twelve meridians connect with the viscera interiorly and link with the limbs exteriorly, diseases can be diagnosed according to the changes of the meridians. For example, cough and asthma can be observed in the disorders of both the lung meridian and the kidney meridian. This is because the kidney meridian runs inside the body and its **longitudinal** part runs **transversely** from the kidney, through the liver and to the lung. So insufficiency of kidney *qi* or invasion of pathogenic factors into the kidney can also bring about cough and asthma. However, there are still some differences between the kidney meridian and lung meridian in causing cough and asthma. Generally speaking, cough and asthma due to the disorder of the lung meridian are accompanied by symptoms of lung distension, chest distress and pain in the **supraclavicular** fossa; while cough and asthma due to the disorder of kidney meridian are accompanied by symptoms of suspending sensation of the heart③ and **susceptibility** to fright④.

7　The following are the common clinical manifestations of the disorders of the twelve meridians. The lung meridian: lung distension, cough, asthma, chest distress and fullness, supraclavicular pain, pain or cold sensation in the shoulders and back, spontaneous sweating and pain in the anterior border of the arm.

8　The large intestine meridian: toothache, neck swelling, sore-throat, yellowish eyes, dry mouth, **epistaxis**, pain in the anterior part of the shoulder and the index finger.

9　The stomach meridian: nasal pain, epistaxis, toothache, facial **distortion**, pain of the **pharynx**, swelling and pain of the knee as well as pain around the breast, thigh, **lateral** part of the leg,

---

　①　According to the theory of meridian system, musculature zones form a system through which *qi* from the twelve meridians "retains, accumulates, disperses and connects" in the musculature and joints: 根据经络学说，经筋是十二经脉之气"结、聚、散、络"于筋肉、关节的体系。
　②　Similarly, when the pathological changes have taken place in the viscera, they may be transmitted to the surface of the body through the system of meridians: 同样，当脏腑发生病变时，也会通过经脉反映于体表。
　③　suspending sensation of the heart: 心悬若饥。
　④　susceptibility to fright: 善恐，病证名。

dorsum of foot and middle toe.

10　The spleen meridian: stiff tongue①, postcibal vomiting, stomachache, abdominal distension, frequent sighing, heavy sensation of the body, inability to move the body, **dysphagia**, **dysphoria**, acute pain below the heart, loose stool②, abdominal mass, diarrhea, retention of urine③, **jaundice**, inability to sleep and flaccidity of the big toe.

11　The heart meridian: dry mouth, heart pain, thirst with desire for drinking, yellowish eyes, hypochondriac pain, pain in the posterior medial side of the upper arm and feverish pain in the palms.

12　The small intestine meridian: sore-throat, swelling of the **mandible**, inability to move the head, breaking pain of the shoulder and upper arm, deafness, yellowish eyes, swollen neck and pain in the neck, mandible, shoulder, upper arm, elbow and posterior lateral side of the arm.

13　The bladder meridian: chills and fever, stuffy nose and headache; severe pain of eyes, neck, spine and waist; inability to bend the thigh, stiffness of **popliteal** fossa and flaccidity of the small toe.

14　The kidney meridian: hunger without desire for food④, cough with blood in the sputum, **dyspnea**, suspending sensation in the heart, susceptibility to fright, hot sensation in the mouth, dry tongue, swollen throat, sore-throat, **vexation**, heart pain, pain in the spine and posterior medial side of the thigh, flaccidity, somnolence and feverish pain in the sole.

15　The pericardium meridian: feverish palms, spasm of the elbow and arm, swelling of **armpit**, even fullness of the chest⑤, reddish cheeks, yellowish eyes, constant laughing, vexation and heart pain.

16　The triple energizer meridian: deafness, heart and hypochondriac pain, swelling and pain of the throat, sweating and severe pain of eyes; pain of the cheeks, the region behind the ears, shoulder, upper arm, elbow and lateral side of the arm; flaccidity of the small finger and index finger.

17　The gallbladder meridian: bitter taste in the mouth, heart and hypochondriac pain; headache, mandibular pain, supraclavicular pain and swelling, swelling of the armpit, and pain in the chest, hypochondrium, thigh, knee and various joints.

18　The liver meridian: severe lumbago, even dry throat, chest fullness, vomiting, diarrhea, **inguinal hernia**, **enuresis**, retention of urine and lower abdominal swelling in women. (1,216 words)

New Words and Expressions

reticular /rɪˈtɪkjʊlə/ *adj*. forming or covered with a netlike pattern of squares and lines 网状的

weave /wiːv/ *v*. to put many different ideas, subjects, stories etc. together and connect them smoothly 构成

---

①　stiff tongue: 舌强,病证名。舌体伸缩不利的征象。见于外感热病热入心包、内伤杂病之中风证,亦可由热盛伤津或痰浊壅阻所致。

②　loose stool: 便溏,是指大便不成形,形似溏泥,俗称薄粪。

③　retention of urine: 尿潴留,是指膀胱内充满尿液而不能正常排出。按其病史、特点分急性尿潴留和慢性尿潴留两类。

④　hunger without desire for food: 饥不欲食,病证名,指感觉饥饿而又不想进食。

⑤　fullness of the chest: 胸满,病证名。胸部胀满不适,因风寒、热壅、停饮、气滞、血瘀等所致。

conception /kən'sepʃn/ *n*. the process by which a woman or female animal becomes pregnant, or the time when this happens 受孕

thoroughfare /'θʌrəfeə(r)/ *n*. the main road through a place such as a city or village 大道,通衢

musculature /'mʌskjələtʃə(r)/ *n*. system of muscles 肌肉系统

longitudinal /lɒŋgɪ'tjuːdɪnl/ *adj*. of or relating to longitude or length 纵长的

transverse /'trænzvɜːs/ *adj*. crossing from side to side; athwart; crossways 横向的

supraclavicular /sjuːprəklæ'vɪkjʊlə/ *adj*. above the clavicular 锁骨上的

susceptibility /səˌseptə'bɪlətɪ/ *n*. someone's feelings, especially when they are easily offended or upset 易感性,敏感性

epistaxis /epɪ'stæksɪs/ *n*. nosebleed 鼻衄

distortion /dɪ'stɔːʃn/ *n*. twisting out of natural, usual, or original shape or condition 扭曲;变形;反常

pharynx /'færɪŋks/ *n*. the tube that goes from the back of your mouth to the place where the tube divides for food and air 咽

lateral /'lætərəl/ *adj*. relating to the sides of something, or movement to the side 侧面的;横(向)的

dorsum /'dɔːsəm/ *n*. back 背部

dysphagia /dɪs'feɪdʒɪə/ *n*. difficulty in swallowing 吞咽困难

dysphoria /dɪs'fɔːrɪə/ *n*. restlessness 烦躁不安

jaundice /'dʒɔːndɪs/ *n*. a medical condition in which your skin and the white part of your eyes become yellow 黄疸

mandible /'mændɪbl/ *n*. the jaw bone of an animal or fish, especially the lower jaw 颌,尤指下颌

popliteal /pɒ'plɪtɪəl/ *adj*. of, relating to, or near the part of the leg behind the knee 腘的

dyspnea /dɪs'pniːə/ *n*. difficulty in breathing 呼吸困难

vexation /vek'seɪʃn/ *n*. the feeling, fact, or state of being vexed; displeasure 烦恼;苦恼;伤脑筋;折磨

armpit /'ɑːmpɪt/ *n*. the hollow place under the arm at the shoulder 腋窝

inguinal /'ɪŋgwɪn(ə)l/ *adj*. of groin 腹股沟的

hernia /'hɜːnɪə/ *n*. a medical condition in which an organ pushes through the muscles that are supposed to contain it 疝气

enuresis /enjʊə'riːsɪs/ *n*. a medical condition of involuntary discharge of urine, especially during sleep 遗尿

FOLLOW-UP ACTIVITIES

Task One   Comprehension Check

1. Questions for Discussion

1) In which meridian can cough and asthma be observed? Why?

2) Please summarize the differences between the kidney meridian and lung meridian in causing cough and asthma.

3) What are the common clinical manifestations of the lung meridian disorders?

4) Please list the meridians which are related to yellowish eyes.

5) When patients suffer from bitter taste in the mouth, what kind of meridian disorder she/he might have?

2. Chart Completion

Meridian system, whose theory focuses on the study of 1) _____ and 2) _____ of human body as a whole, is the foundation for 3) _____, moxibustion, Tuina and Qigong. It refers to the pathways for *qi* to circulate in the body, linking the upper part of the body with the lower part and the interior portion with the exterior.

To better understand this system, the following chart may be of help.

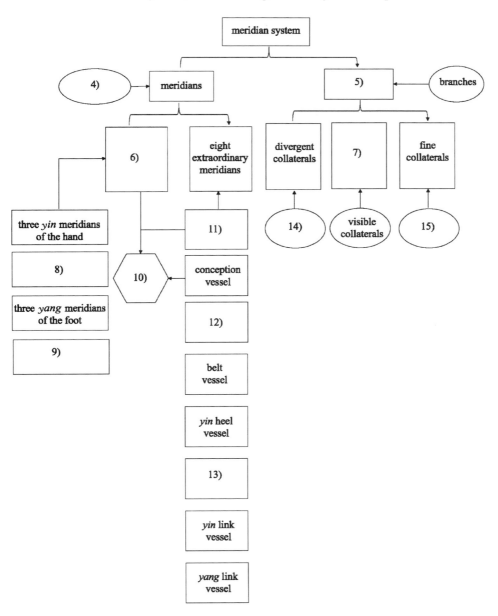

1) _____ 2) _____ 3) _____ 4) _____ 5) _____
6) _____ 7) _____ 8) _____ 9) _____ 10) _____
11) _____ 12) _____ 13) _____ 14) _____ 15) _____

Task Two   Vocabulary

1. Directions: Complete the following phrases respectively according to its corresponding meaning or equivalent in Chinese within the brackets.

1) _____ （任脉）

2) _____ （督脉）

3) _____ （易感性）to fright

4) _____ （软弱无力）of the big toe

5) the_____ （后内侧）side of the thigh

6) form a large_____ （环状物）

7) _____ （热痛）in the palms

8) _____ （食后）vomiting

9) _____ （阳维）vessel

10) twelve_____ （经筋）

11) the_____ （连属部分）of the twelve regular meridians

12) _____ （自发的）sweating

13) _____ （冲脉）

14) _____ （入侵）of pathogenic factors

15) lung_____ （胀）

16) chest _____ （闷）

17) _____ （侧面的）part of the leg

18) facial _____ （扭曲）

19) _____ （三）energizer

20) _____ （腹部的）distension

21) _____ （纵长的）part

22) _____ （季肋）pain

23) _____ （充当）the pathways

24) _____ （不能）to sleep

25) _____ （善恐）

26) _____ （别）collaterals

27) _____ （悬浮）sensation of the heart

28) _____ （表里）relation

29) twelve skin _____ （部门）

30) the_____ （浅表）regions

2. Match the following words with their proper meanings.

Column I	Column II
1) subsidiary	a. (of a part of the body) at or near the front
2) divergent	b. the bottom surface of the foot
3) superficial	c. the finger next to the thumb
4) longitudinal	d. an anatomical depression, trench, or hollow area
5) transverse	e. of or relating to longitude or length
6) sole	f. located behind sth. or at the back of sth.
7) portion	g. mutually joined or related
8) interconnect	h. diverging or causing divergence
9) fossa	i. the fact of not being able to do sth.
10) anterior	j. the main road through a place such as a city or village
11) inability	k. less important than but related or supplementary to
12) posterior	l. pain in the muscles and joints of the lower back
13) thoroughfare	m. existing or occurring at or on the surface
14) index finger	n. one part of sth. larger
15) lumbago	o. crossing from side to side; athwart; crossways

3. Fill in the blanks with the words from the box and change the form when necessary.

interconnected	susceptibility	lumbago	loop	respectively
posterior	transverse	subsidiary	divergent	anterior
inability	index finger	portion	fossa	longitudinal

1) The increased volume was found in the _____ , or front part, of the hippocampus (海马体).

2) Every few weeks, I saw Hannah jogging in _____ around the park.

3) According to Winchester Hospital, a _____ process fracture (横突骨折) is a break in the wing-like bones on side of each vertebra (椎骨) in the spine.

4) The field of psychology is rich with _____ studies, going back to 1946, when the United Kingdom's Medical Research Council began a survey of more than 5,000 people from birth to old age.

5) Regional officials were criticized for their slow response and their _____ to stop similar attacks.

6) Wallinga says he's least confident about the _____ of each age group to infection and the rate at which people of various ages transmit the virus.

7) Any affection involving discomfort, pain, ache, or disability of the large muscles in the

lumbar regions is likely to be called _____, not only by patients but by physicians.

8) Their _____ approaches to the president's signature campaign issue speak to more than the ideological gulf (分歧) between the two men.

9) "It's often initially thought to be a back issue, because the fracture occurs on the _____ side of the body," Simpson says.

10) Two of those accusers (指控者), Jane Doe III and Jane Doe IV, were 13 and 15 years old _____, when they met Epstein.

11) Part of that is following up on complaints we receive about unlicensed shops, and a pretty large _____ of the unlicensed shops happen to be in Southern California.

12) A "_____" is a cavity or depression in the surface.

13) But it's not enough to simply rebuild our roads and fix our bridges; we need to reinvest in a modern, _____ transportation network for future generations.

14) Goldstein was wounded in both hands and lost the _____ on his right hand in the shooting.

15) This is a _____ flue (烟道) of the main chimney.

Task Three　Translation

1　Translate the following medical expressions into English

1) 经络系统
2) 十二正经
3) 奇经八脉
4) 经脉
5) 阳维脉
6) 十五别络
7) 络脉
8) 结、聚、散、络
9) 脾之大络
10) 经络之气
11) 寒战发热
12) 便溏
13) 舌僵
14) 口苦
15) 肾气虚
16) 善太息
17) 身重
18) 邪气
19) 肺经失调
20) 活血通络

2　Translate the following sentences into Chinese or English

1) Meridian system is the most important part of TCM. It serves as the foundation for acupuncture, moxibustion, Tuina and Qigong.

2) These pathways connect the viscera with the limbs and joints, link the upper part of the body with the lower part and associate the interior portion with the exterior.

3) The meridians run in order and interconnect as a large loop while the collaterals run reticularly to weave all the viscera, organs, orifices, muscles, skin and bones of the body.

4) The meridians are the major trunks in this system while the collaterals are the branches of the meridians.

5) Generally speaking, cough and asthma due to the disorder of lung meridian are accompanied by symptoms of lung distension, chest distress and pain in the supraclavicular fossa; while

cough and asthma due to the disorder of kidney meridian are accompanied by symptoms of suspending sensation of the heart and susceptibility to fright.

6）经络学说是研究人体经络的生理功能、病理变化及其与脏腑相互关系的学说。（physiological, pathological）

7）络脉可分为三类，即别络、浮络和孙络。（be divided into ...）

8）别络是最大且主要的络脉，其主要功能是加强经脉表里上的联系。（exterior and interior relation）

9）在发生病变时，经络就成为传递病邪和反映病变的途径。（transmit）

10）临床上将疾病症状出现的部位，结合经络循环的部位和所联系的脏腑，作为疾病诊断的依据。（serve as）

3   Translate the following passage into English

《黄帝内经》分为两部书，其中之一称为《灵枢经》，也称为《针经》，就是专门论述用微针治疗经络的著作。《黄帝内经》对经络做了系统的总结，在经脉之外，增加了络脉、经别、经筋、皮部和奇经等新的概念，它们共同组成了经络系统，成为古人心目中人体最重要的生理结构。

 Text B

Tuina Massage

1   Originated in ancient China, Tuina or *tuina* massage is believed to be the oldest system of bodywork. It's one of the four main branches of traditional Chinese medicine, along with acupuncture, *Qigong*, and Chinese herbal medicine. Through the application of massage and manipulation techniques, *tuina* seeks to establish a more harmonious flow of *qi* through the meridian system, allowing the body to naturally heal itself. Tuina stimulates the flow of *qi* to promote balance and harmony within the body. It's similar to acupuncture in the way it targets specific acupoints, but *tuina* practitioners use fingers instead of needles to apply pressure to stimulate these acupoints.

2   The philosophy and principles of *tuina* massage are based on traditional Chinese medicine, which focuses on emotional and physical components of a person's well-being, as well as aspects such as climate, relationships and diet. Health problems occur when the flow of *qi* is blocked at any acupoint along a meridian (an invisible line that connects your organs with other parts of your body). Similar to acupuncture, *tuina* massage uses the same energetic meridians and acupoints to balance *qi* and blood in a person's body by getting rid of blockages and disturbances that

manifest as illness, disease, and emotional issues. The underlying philosophy of *tuina* massage is that true health is achieved when one has found harmony and balance inside the self and their environment. The main therapeutic goal of *tuina* massage is to remove the energetic blocks that are causing *qi* stagnation.

3   During a session, practitioners use **oscillating** and pressure techniques that differ in force and speed. Tuina massage can be done as a stronger deep-tissue massage or a more gentle, energetic treatment. The practitioner massages the muscles and tendons and uses manipulation techniques to realign the body. Depending on your practitioner as well as your specific needs, various techniques will be used in a session. Passive joint movements are used to restore function to muscles and joints. To enhance the effects of the treatment, herbal **poultices**, **compresses**, **liniments**, and **salves** are used. Tuina massage uses techniques such as **acupressure**, **myofascial** release, and **reflexology**. Sometimes, techniques that are common to **osteopathy** and **chiropractic**, such as stretching and joint **mobilizations**, are also used. There are eight basic techniques used in *tuina* massage:

- **palpating**,
- rejoining,
- opposing,
- lifting,
- pressing,
- **kneading**,
- pushing,
- holding.

Other techniques include:

- Rolling. This is used for injuries such as sprains and strains.
- One-finger technique. This is one-finger stimulation of acupressure points.
- Nei gung. This is a full-body manipulation technique.

4   Tuina massage can be used to treat pain and illness, or to maintain good health. The technique is effective in reducing stress, encouraging relaxation, and deepening sleep. It's often used for conditions and injuries related to the **musculoskeletal** and nervous systems. Here are some common problems *tuina* massage can treat:

- neck and back pain

oscillate /ˈɒsɪleɪt/ *v.* 振荡；摆动

poultice /ˈpəʊltɪs/ *n.* 泥敷剂

compress /kəmˈpres/ *n.* 敷贴

liniment /ˈlɪnəmənt/ *n.* 搽剂

salve /sælv/ *n.* 软膏

acupressure /ˈækjupreʃə(r)/ *n.* 针压法

myofascial /maɪɔːˈfæʃl/ *adj.* 肌筋膜的

reflexology /ˈriːfleksˈɒlədʒɪ/ *n.* 反射疗法

osteopathy /ˌɒstɪˈɒpəθɪ/ *n.* 整骨疗法

chiropractic /ˌkaɪərəʊˈpræktɪk/ *n.* 脊椎按摩疗法

mobilization /ˌməʊbɪlaɪˈzeɪʃn/ *n.* 松动术，活动

palpate /pælˈpeɪt/ *v.* 触摸

kneading /ˈniːdɪŋ/ *n.* 揉捏法

musculoskeletal /ˌmʌskjʊləʊˈskelɪt(ə)l/ *adj.* 肌骨骼的

- musculoskeletal disorders
- premenstrual syndrome
- fatigue and insomnia
- **carpal tunnel**
- **sciatica**
- **migraine**
- **fibromyalgia**
- headaches
- arthritis
- **osteoporosis**
- stress
- digestive conditions
- **respiratory** conditions

5   While some of the research is **preliminary** and ongoing, there's plenty of evidence to back the effectiveness of *tuina* massage in treating health conditions. Some studies indicate that *tuina* massage can successfully：

- **boost** and invigorate the flow of *qi* and blood；
- expel, clear, and **dissipate** pathogenic factors；
- regulate *qi* and blood；
- harmonize *yin* and *yang*；
- improve and regulate the functions of the internal organs；
- release and relax the channel sinews；
- lubricate and facilitate the movement of joints.

6   Let's see what some of the studies say about the benefits in detail. A 2018 study found that *tuina* massage combined with a Chinese medicine foot bath was therapeutically beneficial for people with early-stage diabetic foot. People who received *tuina* massage and a foot bath in addition to **conventional** medicine showed significant improvements compared to people who received only conventional medicine. Another study shows that *tuina* massage is a viable option for people with cancer who want to manage symptoms related to the disease and its conventional treatment. A 2016 meta-analysis assessed the effect of *tuina* massage on improving symptoms and quality of life for people with cancer. When combined with acupuncture, *tuina* massage was effective in improving the quality of life in people with **terminal** cancer. Though *tuina* massage shows promise as a therapy to treat people with cancer, more in-depth research is needed, as many of

carpal tunnel /ˈkɑːplˈtʌnl/ *n*. 腕道综合征

sciatica /saɪˈætɪkə/ *n*. 坐骨神经痛

migraine /ˈmaɪɡreɪn/ *n*. 偏头痛

fibromyalgia /ˌfaɪbrəʊmaɪˈældʒɪə/ *n*. 纤维肌痛

osteoporosis /ˌɒstɪəʊpəˈrəʊsɪs/ *n*. 骨质疏松症

respiratory /rəˈspɪrətrɪ/ *adj*. 呼吸的

preliminary /prɪˈlɪmɪnərɪ/ *adj*. 初步的

boost /buːst/ *v*. 促进

dissipate /ˈdɪsɪpeɪt/ *v*. 使消散

conventional /kənˈvenʃənl/ *adj*. 常规的

terminal /ˈtɜːmɪnl/ *adj*. 晚期的

the studies had limitations.

7   Tuina massage is a safe treatment and is generally well-tolerated. However, remember that it's not a gentle or relaxing massage, and you may feel some discomfort during or after a session. Slight bruising is possible. It's not recommended for people who have fractures or are prone to fractures, vein **inflammation**, or any type of open wound. It's also not recommended for people with previous chronic back issues, such as **ankylosing spondylitis**.

8   When you see a doctor, talk to him or her before adding *tuina* massage to your treatment plan if you have any health concerns. Your doctor may recommend that you use *tuina* massage as a complement to conventional treatment. Additionally, they may recommend another **alternative** treatment to be used alongside *tuina* massage. If you experience any adverse effects or changes to your condition after a *tuina* treatment, talk to your doctor.

9   Tuina massage is a healing technique that offers an **array** of benefits. If you're interested in trying it, contact a certified practitioner. As with many healing **modalities**, *tuina* massage works well when combined with other natural treatments and a healthy lifestyle. Your practitioner may encourage you to do self-massage, stretches, and exercises on your own to increase the benefits of each treatment. (953 words)

(Adapted from https：// www.healthline.com/health/tuina ♯ how-it-works)

inflammation /ˌɪnfləˈmeɪʃn/ *n*. 炎症；发炎
ankylosing spondylitis /ˌæŋkɪˈləuzɪŋˌspɒndɪˈlaitɪs/ *n*. 强直性脊柱炎

alternative /ɔːlˈtɜːnətɪv/ *adj*. 替代性的

array /əreɪ/ *n*. 一系列

modality /məʊˈdælətɪ/ *n*. 方法；疗法

Notes：

1. Through the application of massage and manipulation techniques, *tuina* seeks to establish a more harmonious flow of *qi* through the meridian system, allowing the body to naturally heal itself. 通过运用按摩和一些手法与技巧，旨在促进气在经络之中循行畅通，使人体自愈。

2. Similar to acupuncture, *tuina* massage uses the same energetic meridians and acupoints to balance *qi* and blood in a person's body by getting rid of blockages and disturbances that manifest as illness, disease, and emotional issues. 与针灸治疗类似，推拿也作用于经络和穴位，以调和气血，消除疾病和情绪不畅等人体失调和紊乱问题。

3. To enhance the effects of the treatment, herbal poultices, compresses, liniments, and salves are used. 有时推拿与草药泥敷剂、敷贴、搽剂和软膏配合使用，以提高疗效。

4. myofascial release 筋膜放松疗法，缩写为 MFR，是一种替代药物的疗法，可用于治疗肌筋膜疼痛综合征（myofascial pain syndrome, MPS）。

5. Sometimes, techniques that are common to osteopathy and chiropractic, such as stretching and joint mobilizations, are also used. 有时，也使用诸如拉伸法和关节松动术等整骨疗法和脊椎指

压疗法这类常见手法。

6. There are eight basic techniques used in *tuina* massage: palpating, rejoining, opposing, lifting, pressing, kneading, pushing, holding. 推拿有八种基本手法：摸法、接法、端法、提法、按法、摩法、推法、拿法。

7. One-finger technique 一指禅法，以一指禅推法为主要手法来防治疾病的推拿方法。"一指禅"是佛教禅宗用语，意为万物归一。

8. Nei gung 内功法推拿疗法是以擦法为主要手法，并指导患者进行少林内功锻炼，以防治疾病的一种推拿疗法。

9. musculoskeletal disorders 肌骨失常

10. premenstrual syndrome 经前综合征，常使用缩写 PMS。

11. While some of the research is preliminary and ongoing, there's plenty of evidence to back the effectiveness of *tuina* massage in treating health conditions. 虽然部分研究尚处于初级阶段，仍在进行之中，但是有大量证据显示推拿在治疗疾病方面是有效的。

12. channel sinews 经筋

13. lubricate and facilitate the movement of joints 滑利关节

14. A 2018 study found that *tuina* massage combined with a Chinese medicine foot bath was therapeutically beneficial for people with early-stage diabetic foot. 2018 年的一项研究发现，推拿结合中药足浴对早期糖尿病足患者疗效显著。

15. conventional treatment 常规治疗

16. A 2016 meta-analysis assessed the effect of *tuina* massage on improving symptoms and quality of life for people with cancer. 2016 年的一项分析对推拿改善癌症患者症状和生活质量的效果进行了评估。

17. It's not recommended for people who have fractures or are prone to fractures, vein inflammation, or any type of open wound. 建议有骨折或容易骨折、静脉炎或其他开放性伤口的患者不要使用推拿疗法。

18. alternative treatment 替代疗法

19. adverse effects 不良反应

Task One　Reading Comprehension

1. What is the main therapeutic goal of *tuina* massage? _____
   A. To release and relax the channel sinews
   B. To regulate *qi* and blood
   C. To remove the energetic blocks that are causing *qi* stagnation.
   D. To expel, clear, and dissipate pathogenic factors

2. _____ is **NOT** a basic technique used in *tuina* massage.
   A. Rolling　　B. Palpating　　C. Pressing　　D. Holding

3. A certified practitioner can use *tuina* together with _____ to improve the quality of life for people with terminal cancer.
   A. cupping　　　　B. spooning

C. Chinese herbal medicine　　　　　D. acupuncture

4. Tuina massage can't treat the following problems **EXCEPT** _____ .

　　A. vein inflammation　　　　　　　B. migraine

　　C. open wound　　　　　　　　　　D. ankylosing spondylitis

5. Which of the following statements about *tuina* is **NOT TRUE**? _____

　　A. There may be some adverse effects or changes to patients' condition after a *tuina* treatment.

　　B. Tuina massage works well when combined with other natural treatments and a healthy lifestyle.

　　C. By stimulating the flow of *qi*, *tuina* massage can promote balance and harmony within the body.

　　D. The oscillating and pressure techniques used during a session are same in force and speed.

Task Two　Vocabulary

1. Directions: Complete the following phrases respectively according to its corresponding meaning or equivalent in Chinese within the brackets.

1) _____ (手法) techniques　　　　2) vein _____ (炎症)

3) _____ (使消散) pathogenic factors　　4) joint _____ (松动术)

5) sprains and _____ (拉伤)　　　　6) slight_____ (瘀伤)

7) _____ (呼吸的) conditions　　　　8) _____ (初步的) research

9) _____ (肌骨骼的) disorders　　　10) _____ (滑利) the movement of joints

11) Chinese medicine _____ (足浴)　12) _____ (常规的) medicine

13) _____ (晚期的) cancer　　　　　　14) channel _____ (筋)

15) specific _____ (穴位)　　　　　16) _____ (整骨疗法) and chiropractic

17) _____ (替代性的) treatment　　18) be _____ (易于遭受) to fractures

19) _____ (不良的) effects　　　　　20) healing _____ (方法)

2. Fill in the blanks with the words from the box and change the form when necessary.

lubricate	dissipate	realign	energetic	premenstrual
disturbance	viable	adverse	diabetic	bruising
inflammation	complement	assess	prone	alternative

1) _____ medicine uses traditional ways of curing people, such as medicines made from plants, massage, and acupuncture.

2) Over the weekend, a Florida man hospitalized with the coronavirus claimed hydroxychloroquine (羟氯喹) saved his life, and that his fever and pain _____ soon after the drug was administered.

3) Mountain gorillas are _____ to some respiratory illnesses that afflict (折磨) humans.

4) The fungi is meant to _____ , not replace, traditional cancer treatments such as chemotherapy, she notes.

5) The drug can cause _____ of the liver.

6) Such symptoms include fatigue, headaches, nausea and vomiting, excessive thirst, dizziness or shakiness and mood _____ , among others.

7) Less than four months after the first genetic sequence was published, teams across the world are using open data sharing to develop a _____ vaccine, effective therapeutics and rapid diagnostics.

8) This drug is known to have _____ effects.

9) In my day-to-day work, I routinely _____ which patients require ventilator (呼吸机) support, working with a dedicated team of nurses, pharmacists, respiratory therapists, physical therapists and others, to provide care.

10) She had quite severe _____ and a cut lip.

11) Many women suffer from _____ syndrome, causing headaches and depression.

12) He is an insulin-dependent _____ .

13) When the city of Gothenberg in Sweden introduced a six-hour day for some nurses, the nurses became healthier, happier and more _____ .

14) But in more severe cases, surgery may be recommended to _____ the bone, ligament, tendon and nerves, so that the big toe is brought back to the correct position.

15) Taking several doses of fish oil per day will help to reduce inflammation in the body but also help cleanse your colon (结肠) by _____ your intestinal system.

Task Three   Writing

Please rewrite the text in a form of abstract (about 150 words).

Terminology

Basic Terminology of the Meridian System

Terminology	WHO	WFCMS
经络	meridian and collateral	meridian/channel and collateral
经络现象	meridian phenomenon	meridian/collateral phenomenon
经气;经络之气	meridian *qi*	meridian/collateral *qi*
经络学说	meridian and collateral theory	meridian/channel and collateral theory
经脉	meridian vessel	meridian; channel
循经感传	transmission of sensation along meridian	sensation transmission along meridian/channel
手三阴经	three *yin* meridians of the hand	three *yin* meridians/channels of hand

continued

Terminology	WHO	WFCMS
手三阳经	three *yang* meridians of the hand	three *yang* meridians/channels of hand
足三阳经	three *yang* meridians of the foot	three *yang* meridian/channels of foot
足三阴经	three *yin* meridians of the foot	three *yin* meridians/channels of foot
十四经;十四经脉	fourteen meridians	fourteen meridians/channels
十二经;十二正经;十二经脉	twelve meridians	twelve meridians/channels
奇经	extra meridian	extra meridian/channel
奇经八脉	eight extra meridians	eight extra meridians/channels
督脉	governor vessel (GV)	governor vessel (GV)
任脉	conception vessel (CV)	conception vessel (CV)
冲脉	thoroughfare vessel	thoroughfare vessel (TV)
带脉	belt vessel	belt vessel (BV)
阴跷脉	*yin* heel vessel	*yin* heel vessel (*Yin* HV)
阳跷脉	*yang* heel vessel	*yang* heel vessel (*Yang* HV)
阴维脉	*yin* link vessel	*yin* link vessel (*Yin* LV)
阳维脉	*yang* link vessel	*yang* link vessel (*Yang* LV)
十二经别	twelve meridian divergences	twelve meridian/channel divergences
经别	meridian divergence	meridian/channel divergence
十二经筋	twelve meridian sinews	twelve meridian/channel sinews
经筋	meridian sinew	meridian/channel sinew
十二皮部	twelve cutaneous regions	twelve cutaneous regions
皮部	cutaneous region	cutaneous region
络脉	collateral vessel	collateral vessel
十五络脉	fifteen collateral vessels	fifteen collateral vessels
孙络	tertiary collateral vessel	tertiary collateral vessels
浮络	superficial collateral vessel	superficial collateral vessel
手太阴肺经	lung meridian (LU)	lung meridian/channel of hand greater *yin* (LU); hand greater *yin* lung meridian/channel
手阳明大肠经	large intestine meridian (LI)	large intestine meridian/channel of hand *yang* brightness (LI); hand *yang* brightness large intestine meridian/channel
足阳明胃经	stomach meridian (ST)	stomach meridian/channel of foot *yang* brightness (ST); foot *yang* brightness stomach meridian/channel
足太阴脾经	spleen meridian (SP)	spleen meridian/channel of foot greater *yin* (SP); foot greater *yin* spleen meridian/channel

continued

Terminology	WHO	WFCMS
手少阴心经	heart meridian (HT)	heart meridian/channel of hand lesser *yin* (HT); hand lesser *yin* heart meridian/channel
手太阳小肠经	small intestine meridian (SI)	small intestine meridian/channel of hand greater *yang* (SI); hand greater *yang* small intestine meridian/channel
足太阳膀胱经	bladder meridian (BL)	bladder meridian/channel of foot greater *yang* (BL); foot greater *yang* bladder meridian/channel
足少阴肾经	kidney meridian (KI)	kidney meridian/channel of foot lesser *yin* (KI); foot lesser *yin* kidney meridian/channel
手厥阴心包经	pericardium meridian (PC)	pericardium meridian/ channel of hand reverting *yin* (PC); hand reverting *yin* pericardium meridian/channel
手少阳三焦经	triple energizer meridian (TE)	triple energizer meridian/ channel of hand lesser *yang* (TE); hand lesser *yang* triple energizer meridian/channel
足少阳胆经	gallbladder meridian (GB)	gallbladder meridian/ channel of foot lesser *yang* (GB); foot lesser *yang* gallbladder meridian/channel
足厥阴肝经	liver meridian (LR)	liver meridian/channel of foot reverting *yin* (LR); foot reverting *yin* liver meridian/channel
正经	main meridian	regular meridian/channel
气街	*qi* thoroughfare	① *qi* pathway ② another name for Qichong (ST 30)
鼻衄	nosebleed	epistaxis
肺胀	lung distention	lung distension
喘	dyspnea	dyspnea
咳嗽	cough	cough
胸胁苦满	fullness in the chest and hypochondrium	fullness and discomfort in chest and hypochondrium
喉痹	throat impediment	pharyngitis
便溏	sloppy stool	loose stool
遗尿	enuresis	enuresis
飧泄	swill diarrhea	lienteric diarrhea
推拿	massage	*tuina*; massage
摇法	rocking manipulation	rotating manipulation
一指禅推法	*qi*-concentrated single-finger pushing manipulation	one-finger-pushing manipulation
滚法	rolling manipulation	rolling manipulation
揉法	kneading manipulation	kneading manipulation
摩法	rubbing manipulation	rubbing manipulation

continued

Terminology	WHO	WFCMS
擦法	scrubbing manipulation	scrubbing manipulation
推法	pushing manipulation	pushing manipulation
搓法	twisting manipulation	twisting manipulation
抖法	shaking manipulation	shaking manipulation
按法	pressing manipulation	pressing manipulation
捏法	pinching manipulation	pinching manipulation
拿法	grasping manipulation	grasping manipulation
踩蹻法	treading manipulation	treading manipulation
叩击法	tapping examination	tapping manipulation
弹法	flicking manipulation	flicking manipulation
背法	back-packing manipulation	back-carrying manipulation
扳法	pulling manipulation	pulling manipulation

本书配套数字教学资源

微信扫描二维码，加入中医英语
读者交流圈，获取配套教学视
频、学习课件、课后习题和沟通交
流平台等板块内容，夯实基础知识

Acrid flavor enters the qi. If one consumes too much of it，
this will cause emptiness of his heart.
辛走气，多食之，令人洞心①。

Unit 8　Chinese Materia Medica

Warming-up

Before you listen (Watch)

In this section you will hear a short passage about "Fantastic Herbal Medicine". The following words and phrases may be of help.

cobra /ˈkəʊbrə/	*n.*	眼镜蛇
spring out	*v.*	(从隐蔽处)突然冒出
clan /klæn/	*n.*	宗族；部落
usage /ˈjuːsɪdʒ/	*n.*	使用；用法
potency /ˈpəʊtnsɪ/	*n.*	效能
renowned /rɪˈnaʊnd/	*a.*	著名的
distribute /dɪˈstrɪbjuːt/	*v.*	散布

While you listen(Watch)

Listen to the passage carefully and fill in each of the blanks marked from 1) to 10) according to what you have heard.

Oh my God. Two hundred cobra snakes have escaped from a village near Nanjing. Ah, that's so 1) _____. Oh, I am really not the biggest fan of snakes, not a cobra snake. Oh, imagine if you're just walking down the path, and suddenly a cobra just spring out right in front of you. What would you do?

Today I'm searching for the answer to the question. Here in China, there is clan of people who still follow the ancient Shennong, also known as the emperor of Five 2) _____, who was

---

① 《灵枢·五味论》，Paul U. Unschuld 译。

around five thousand years ago. They still 3) _____ much mysterious wisdom from the past. And I'm sure they must know a way to protect themselves from snakes.

So let's go find out what it is. The usage of herbal medicines in China has a history stretching back over thousands of years. There are now over 12,000 different 4) _____ of Chinese herbal medicines, including medicines that come from plants, animals and minerals. As the majorities of medicines are plant-based, Chinese medicine has then also become known as Chinese herbal medicine.

There are some plants that can be used directly after they are picked; however the majority of plants need to be 5) _____ and cured so that toxic elements can be 6) _____ , and the medicinal elements can be 7) _____ to their full potency. And of course, it makes it much easier to 8) _____ and store. Renowned medical researcher Li Shizhen, used the book "Classified Materia Medica" of a thousand years ago as a foundation for creating the 9) _____ work "Compendium of Materia Medica", which was much needed to suit the developing times. The "Compendium of Materia Medica" was first distributed in the now city of Nanjing, three years after the author Li Shizhen's death. The book recorded 1,892 different medical plants and 11,000 10) _____ . And not only just in China, every year more and more medical practitioners from around the world are coming to China to learn the herbal medicine here. The age-old knowledge of the herbal farmers is now becoming understood and appreciated in modern scientific terms all over the globe.

After you listen(Watch)

Please discuss with your partner the following questions and give your presentation to the class.

1) What was Li Shizhen's contribution to Chinese herbal medicine?

2) Please list some sources of Chinese herbal medicines.

3) Can the majority of herbal plants be used directly after they are picked? And why?

4) What are the health benefits and side effects of having Tulsi tea during pregnancy?

Reading

 Text A

BEFORE CLASS

1. Quest for Definition

Directions: Explore online the definitions of the following terms from Text A and prepare a unique one-minute oral presentation for your class.

1) Chinese medicinal herbs

2) functional tendencies

3) processing and preparation

4) meridian tropism

5) toxicity

6) precautions and contraindications

2. Text-based Activities

Directions: Read carefully the part of Text A that corresponds to your task, and then prepare a unique one-minute oral presentation for your class.

PERFORMANCE IN CLASS

Your Task

1) What is Chinese materia medica?

2) Please briefly introduce the four properties and five tastes of Chinese materia medica.

3) What are the functions of the sweet herbs?

4) Can an herb selectively act upon a particular part of the body? Any examples?

5) What is the functional tendency of an herb?

Chinese Materia Medica

1   There is a great variety of Chinese materia medica①, including plants, animal parts and minerals. Among these materials, flowers, herbs and plants are the ones most frequently used, that is why Chinese materia medica is called Chinese **medicinal** herbs②.

2   The Chinese medicinal herbs are characterized by four **properties** (cold, heat, warm and cool) and five tastes (sour, bitter, sweet, acrid or pungent-spicy and salty). These terms describe the therapeutic significance and energetic characteristics of the herbs and their actions. Herbs like Shigao (*Gypsum Fibrostm*), Zhimu (*Rhizoma Anemarrhenae*), Huanglian (*Rhizoma Coptidis*) root and Shengdihuang (fresh *Radix Rehmanniae*), which relieve heat syndromes, are cool or cold in nature. Herbs such as Fuzi (*Radix Aconiti Praeparata*), which relieve cold syndromes are warm or heat in nature. Herbs whose properties are neither cold nor heat are termed **neutral**, such as Fuling (*Poria*).

3   When the taste is not obvious it is known as **bland** or tasteless. Ancient physician discovered that a particular property could induce certain therapeutic effects. Pungent and spicy herbs disperse and promote the circulation of *qi* and invigorate the blood. For instance, Mahuang (*Herba Ephedrae*) relieves exterior syndrome by inducing sweating; Muxiang (*Radix Aucklandiae*)

---

①   materia medica: 本草。

②   Chinese medicinal herbs: 中草药。

promotes the circulation of *qi*; and Honghua (*Flos Carthami*) invigorates the blood.

4　Sweet herbs have the function of tonifying, harmonizing and moderating. For example, Dangshen (*Radix Codonopsis Pilosulae*) **replenishes** *qi*; Shudihuang (prepared *Radix Rehmanniae*) nourishes blood; and Yitang (*Saccharum Granorum*) and Gancao (*Radix Glycyrrhizae*) moderate, stop pain and harmonize the actions of other herbs. Sour herbs bear absorbing and controlling effects. For instance, Shanzhuyu (*Fructus Corni*) and Wuweizi(*Fructus Schisandrae*) stop **seminal emissions** and spontaneous sweating①; and Wubeizi (*Galla Chinensis*) controls diarrhea. Some herbs are **astringent** in nature. Their action is similar to that of the herbs sour in taste. For example, Longgu (*Os Draconis*) and Muli (*Concha Ostreae*) are used for relieving spontaneous sweating; Chishizhi (*Halloysitum Rubrum*) and Shiliupi (*Pericarpium Granati*) for stopping diarrhea; Qianshi (*Semen Euryales*) and Fupenzi (*Fructus Rubi*) for treating nocturnal emissions, frequent urination and **leukorrhea**.

5　Bitter herbs function to reduce and dry. For example, Dahuang (*Radix et Rhizoma Rhei*) is used to move stool and reduce heat; Tinglizi (*Semen Lepidii seu Descurainiae*) can reduce heat in the lungs and soothes asthma; Cangzhu (*Rhizoma Atractylodis*) and Houpo (*Cortex Magnoliae Ojficianalis*) dry and transform turbid dampness; and Huangbai (*Cortex Phellodendri*) and Zhimu (*Rhizoma Anemarrhenae*) dry dampness and clear heat. Salty herbs soften hardness, release hardenings and nodules and purge stool. For example, Mangxiao (*Natrii Sulfas*) is used for **constipation**; and Walengzi (*Concha Arcae*) treats subcutaneous nodules and scrofula.

6　The functional tendencies of herbs are marked by **ascending, descending, floating** and **sinking** ②. Herbs that ascend and float move upward and outward, promote sweating, raise *yang*, cause vomiting and open the orifices. Herbs that descend and sink move downward and inward, conduct *qi* to flow downward, promote urination and defecation, **subdue** *yang* and calm the mind.

7　In general, the functional tendency of an herb is related to its taste, property, quality and processing. Herbs featured by ascending and floating must be pungent and spicy or sweet in taste and warm or heat in property, while herbs characterized by descending and sinking must be bitter, sour or salty in taste and cool or cold in property.

8　Herb parts, such as flowers and leaves, that are light in quality have the actions of ascending and floating; herbs or substances that are heavy in quality, such as seeds, fruits and minerals, have the actions of descending and sinking. In addition, processing and preparation may change the taste and property of the herb and influence its functional tendencies.

9　An herb may selectively act upon a particular part of the body to relieve pathogenic factors in specific meridians and organs. The meridians that a herb enters depend on the corresponding symptoms relieved. For example, Mahuang (*Herba Ephedrae*) promotes sweating, soothes asthma and benefits urination. It is indicated for fever, chills and absence of sweating due to invasion of exogenous pathogenic wind and cold, dysuria, edema and so on. Judged by the above indications

---

①　stop seminal emissions and spontaneous sweating：固精止汗。
②　ascending, descending, floating and sinking：升降浮沉。

and analysis in accordance with the theories of the *zangfu* organs and meridians, it can be determined that this herb may enter the lung and urinary bladder meridians. Dazao (*Fructus Ziziphi Jujubae*) tonifies *qi* in the spleen and stomach. It is indicated for poor appetite and loose stool due to weakness of the spleen and stomach. So it enters the meridian of the spleen and stomach.

10　In the *Chinese Materia Medica*①, the words "toxic, nontoxic, very toxic or slightly toxic" often appear. The toxicity of herbs and substances not only causes symptomatic reactions but also exerts adverse effects on tissues. So no overdose of toxic herbs should be given as it may lead to side effects. Nontoxic herbs are moderate in nature and, generally speaking, do not have side effects. For example, Dazao (*Fructus Ziziphi Jujubae*) and Fuling (*Poria*) are nontoxic herbs, while Fuzi(*Radix Aconiti Praeparata*) and seed of Maqianzi (*Semen Strychni*) are toxic ones.

11　In the application of herbs, two points have to bear in mind. One is the combination of herbs; the other is the precautions and contraindications

12　Two or more herbs are combined to increase or promote their therapeutic effectiveness, to minimize toxicity or side effects, to accommodate complex clinical situations and to alter their actions. Different combinations can cause variations in therapeutic effect.

13　The precautions and contraindications in the application of herbs include the following aspects:

14　The precautions and contraindications in combination: The historical medical literature contraindicates certain herbs and substances. These include the eighteen incompatible medicinal herbs② and the nineteen mutually-restraining medicinal herbs③.

15　The precautions and contraindications during pregnancy: It is contraindicated to prescribe herbs with strong actions or toxicity, especially Badou (*Fructus Crotonis*), Qianniuzi (*Semen Pharbitidis*), Daji (*Radix Euphorbiae Pekinensis*) and Sanleng (*Rhizoma Sparganii*) for pregnant women. Pungent-spicy and hot herbs that promote circulation of *qi* and remove stagnation of *qi* and blood should be used with caution during pregnancy. These include Taoren (*Semen Persicae*), Honghua (*Flos Carthami*), and Fuzi (*Radix Aconiti Praeparata*).

16　The precautions and contraindications in food intake: Certain foods may influence the action of herbs or bring about some abnormalities. It is advisable in general not to eat raw cold, greasy, strong smelling or spicy food while taking medicine. The historical literature records that Changshan (*Radix Dichroae*) is contraindicated with onion; Dihuang (*Radix Rehmanniae*) and Heshouwu (*Radix Polygoni Multiflori*) are contraindicated with onion, garlic and turnip; Bohe (*Herba Menthae*) is contraindicated with turtle meat; Fuling (*Poria*) is contraindicated with vinegar; and Biejia (*Carrapax Trionycis*) is contraindicated with three-colored amaranth.

17　Each herb has its own indications; the clinician should not select herbs at random. He or she

---

①　*Chinese Materia Medica*:《中华本草》。
②　the eighteen incompatible medicinal herbs：十八反。
③　the nineteen mutually-restraining medicinal herbs：十九畏。

must know the properties, tastes and actions of the herbs. For example, Mahuang (*Herba Ephedrae*) is pungent-spicy in taste and warm in property, having the function of inducing sweating. It is used to treat fever, chills and absence of sweating due to an invasion of exogenous wind and cold. It is contraindicated in deficiency exterior syndrome with the symptoms mentioned above. (1,199 words)

New Words and Expressions

medicinal /mə'dısınl/ *adj*. helpful in the process of healing illness or infection 有疗效的;药用的;药的

property /'prɒpətɪ/ *n*. a quality or characteristic that sth has 性质;特性

neutral /'njuːtrəl/ *adj*. supporting or helping either side in a dispute, contest, war, etc.; impartial 中立的;中性的

bland /blænd/ *adj*. not having a strong or interesting taste 淡的

replenish /rɪ'plenɪʃ/ *v*. fill something again; get a further supply for something 补充,使充满精神活力

seminal /'semɪnl/ *adj*. of or containing semen 精液的;含精液的

emission /ɪ'mɪʃən/ *n*. a substance that is emitted or released 排放物;散发物

astringent /ə'strɪndʒənt/ *adj*. having the effect of astringing; styptic 收涩的

leukorrhea /ˌljuːkə'riːə/ *n*. a whitish, viscid discharge from the vagina 白带

constipation /ˌkɒnstɪ'peɪʃn/ *n*. the condition of being unable to get rid of waste material from the bowels easily 便秘

ascend /ə'send/ *v*. to rise; to go up; to climb up 上升;升高;登高

descend /dɪ'send/ *v*. to come or go down from a higher to a lower level 下来;下去;下降

float /fləʊt/ *v*. to move slowly on water or in the air 浮动;漂流;飘动;飘移

sink /sɪŋk/ *v*. to go down below the surface or towards the bottom of a liquid or soft substance 下沉;下陷;沉没

subdue /səb'djuː/ *v*. bring something or somebody under control by force; defeat 克制,抑制,缓和,减轻

toxicity /tɔk'sɪsɪtɪ/ *n*. quality or degree of being toxic 毒性

moderate /'mɔdərɪt/ *adj*. average in amount, intensity, quality, etc. 适度的,温和的; *v*. become less violent, extreme or intense 使和缓,使减轻

incompatible /ˌɪnkəm'pætəbl/ *adj*. (with sth) two actions, ideas, etc. that are incompatible are not acceptable or possible together because of basic differences (与某事物)不一致,不相配

precaution /prɪ'kɔːʃn/ *n*. (against sth) something that is done in advance in order to prevent problems or to avoid danger 预防措施;预防;防备

contraindication /ˌkɒntrəˌɪndɪ'keɪʃn/ *n*. a possible reason for not giving sb. a particular drug or medical treatment (对某种药物或疗法的)禁忌(原因)

vinegar /'vɪnɪgə/ *n*. sour liquid made from malt, wine, cider, etc. by fermentation and used for flavoring food and for pickling 醋

indication /ˌɪndɪ'keɪʃn/ *n*. a symptom or particular circumstance that indicates the advisability or necessity of a specific medical treatment or procedure 适应证

FOLLOW-UP ACTIVITIES

Task one   Comprehension Check

1. Questions for Discussion

1) In the application of herbs, what are the purposes of combining two herbs?

2) What are precautions and contraindications in the application of herbs?

3) What are the differences between Western herbology and Chinese herbology?

4) What are new technologies and methods for identifying traditional Chinese medicinal material?

2. Chart Completion

> **INTRODUCTION: (para. 1)**
>   Chinese materia medica, called 1) _____ includes plants, animal parts and minerals, of which flowers, herbs and plants are the ones most frequently used.
>
> **FOUR PROPERTIES and Five TASTES: (para. 2 – 5)**
>   Four properties refer to 2) _____ and five tastes refer to sour, bitter, sweet, acrid or pungent-spicy and salty flavors. Ancient physician discovered that a particular property could induce certain therapeutic effects.
> ● Pungent and spicy herbs 3) _____.
> ● Sweet herbs have the function of 4) _____.
> ● Sour herbs bear 5) _____.
> ● Bitter herbs function to 6) _____.
> ● Salty herbs function to 7) _____.
> **Functional Tendency: (para. 6 – 8)**
>   The functional tendency of an herb is related to its 8) _____.
> Herb parts, that are light in quality have the actions of 9) _____; herbs or substances that are heavy in quality have the actions of 10) _____.
> **Meridian Tropism and Toxicity**
>   The meridians that an herb enters depend on the corresponding symptoms relieved. For example, Mahuang enters 11) _____:
>   In *Chinese Materia Medica*, the words 12)"_____" often appear.
> **Precautions and Contraindications**
>   The precautions and contraindications in the application of herbs include the following aspects:
>   The precautions and contraindications in combination, 13) _____, and in food intake.

Task Two   Vocabulary

1. Directions: Complete the following phrases respectively according to its corresponding meaning or equivalent in Chinese within the brackets.

1) Chinese_____（药物的）herbs   2) _____（淡味的）herbs

3) _____（缓解）cold syndromes

4) a particular_____（性质）

5) _____（使生气勃勃）the blood

6) _____（调和）the actions of other herbs

7) _____（夜间的）emission

8) soothe _____（哮喘）

9) release hardenings and _____（结节）

10) _____（加工）and preparation

11) _____（功能的）tendency

12) _____（选择性地）act upon

13) benefit _____（排尿）

14) _____（没有）of sweating

15) the _____（经络）of the spleen and stomach

16) slightly _____（有毒的）

17) causes _____（有症状的）reactions

18) exert _____（不良的）effects

19) _____（药量过多）of toxic herbs

20) _____（组合）of herbs

21) _____（改变）their actions

22) _____（相互抑制的）medicinal herbs

23) precautions and _____（禁忌证）

24) _____（开药方）herbs

25) _____（治疗的）effect

26) _____（油腻的）food

27) historical _____（文献）

28) _____（引起）sweating

29) Food _____（摄入）

30) open the _____（孔口）

2. Match the following words with their proper meanings.

Column I	Column II
1) pungent	a. of or relating to or occurring in the night
2) characteristic	b. something is situated, used, or put under your skin
3) therapeutic	c. happening or arising without apparent external cause
4) disperse	d. direct the course of
5) turbid	e. tending to cure or restore to health
6) spontaneous	f. a distinguishing quality
7) nocturnal	g. the state of being pregnant
8) subcutaneous	h. a strong, sharp smell or taste which is often so strong that it is unpleasant
9) conduct	i. make a treatment inadvisable
10) accommodate	j. widely cultivated plant having a large fleshy edible white or yellow root
11) variation	k. a measure taken in advance to ward off impending danger
12) contraindicate	l. distribute loosely
13) pregnancy	m. adapt or make fit for, or change to suit a new purpose
14) turnip	n. (of especially liquids) clouded as with sediment
15) precaution	o. a change or slight difference in a level, amount, or quantity

3. Fill in the blanks with the words from the box and change the form when necessary.

pungent	replenish	medicinal	incompatible	turbid
spontaneous	nocturnal	subcutaneous	conduct	accommodate
variation	contraindicate	pregnancy	turnip	emission

1) The little streamlet, once crystal and sunshine, is now _____ .

2) Green tea's _____ properties are primarily linked to a family of compounds known as catechins (茶多酚).

3) In the U. S. the drug is _____ for patients with a history of heart disease, though prescribers do not always follow such guidelines.

4) Sometimes to _____ cultural and individual needs, the courses are arranged for evenings and weekends.

5) A _____ smell of disinfectant, mixed with the odor of charred (烧焦的) bodies, hung in the air of the hospital.

6) It would be wiser to cut out all alcohol during _____ .

7) We _____ a weekly poll of our members and amplify the results with mainstream media.

8) You need to eat something to _____ nutrients and help your body recover from physical wear and tear (损耗).

9) Whether this is enough to offset the rise in carbon _____ is another matter.

10) The recommendations apply to "planned or _____" events, including conferences, festivals, parades, concerts, sporting events and weddings.

11) Keeping track of immunizations can be challenging in wealthy countries, where electronic health records may be _____ between different health care providers.

12) A _____ is a round vegetable with a greenish-white skin that is the root of a crop.

13) Symptoms reported by local clinicians include high fever, nausea, and vomiting, followed by meningitis (脑膜炎), _____ haemorrhage (出血), toxic shock, and coma in severe cases.

14) The survey found a wide _____ in the prices charged for canteen food.

15) It can cure kidney disease, _____ emission and frequent urination.

Task Three   Translation

1   Translate the following medical expressions into English

1) 中草药

2) 四气五味

3) 补益、和中、缓急

4) 行气活血

5) 炮制

6) 无毒

7) 止泻

8) 发汗解表

9) 收敛固涩

10) 软坚散结

11) 泻热通便

12) 升降沉浮

13) 归经

14) 用药禁忌

15) 燥湿清热

16) 引气下行

17) 平喘利尿

18) 十八反

19) 十九畏

20) 潜阳安神

2   Translate the following sentences into Chinese or English

1) Among these materials, flowers, herbs and trees are the ones most frequently used, that is

why Chinese materia medica is called Chinese medicinal herbs.

2) Herbs that ascend and float move upward and outward; they promote sweating, raise *yang*, cause vomiting and open the orifices.

3) The meridians that an herb enters depend on the corresponding symptoms relieved.

4) No overdose of toxic herbs should be given as this may lead to side effects.

5) Two or more herbs are combined to increase or promote their therapeutic effectiveness and to minimize toxicity or side effects.

6) 中草药具有四气和五味。(be characterized by)

7) 一个药物可以有选择性地作用于人体的某一特定部位以消除某一经络或器官的病变。(act upon)

8) 该药主治脾胃虚弱所致食欲不振、便溏。(be indicated for)

9) 禁止开药效强或有毒性的药物。(be contraindicated)

10) 临床医生不能随意选药。(at random)

3 Translate the following passage into English

《本草纲目》是明代著名的医学家李时珍所著。这部著作近200万字,记载药物1892种。除了中草药,该书也包含了动物和矿物质作为药物的记载。《本草纲目》堪称中医史上最完整的医书,对各种药物的名称、气味、形态等都做了详尽的介绍。它被翻译成20多种语言并在全世界广为流传。即便现在,人们还常常将它用作医学参考书。

Text B

Traditional Chinese Medical Prescriptions

1　The art of prescriptions, also known as **recipes** or formulas, in traditional Chinese herbal medicine has undergone significant change through centuries. Like other aspects of TCM, it is important to understand the nature of this development in order to clearly appreciate how the prescriptions came to be, and how to use them in the clinic to the best effect.

recipe /ˈresɪpɪ/ *n*.(这里指的是)处方;药方

2　The prescriptions in TCM are not merely collections of medicinal substances in which the actions of one herb are simply added to those of another in a **cumulative** fashion. They are complex recipes of interrelated substances, each of which affects the actions of the others in the prescription. It is this complex interaction which makes the prescriptions so effective, but also difficult to study.

cumulative /ˈkjuːmjulətɪv/ *adj*.(数量、力量等)渐增的;积累的

3　Every medicinal substance has its strengths and shortcomings. An effective prescription is one in which the substances are carefully balanced to **accentuate** the strengths and reduce the side-effects. The combination of substances in a prescription creates a new therapeutic agent that can treat diseases much more effectively than a single substance.

4   Constructing an effective prescription involves more than simply putting ingredients together to obtain a certain effect. One needs a principle to guide the construction so that the ingredients are combined in an **optimal** fashion. The orderly arrangement of ingredients in a prescription is called a **hierarchy**. Traditional Chinese society was always very conscious of rank, which revolved in the first instance around the emperor and his court. For this reason, the terms used to signify the importance or rank of the ingredients in a prescription reflect those used at court. The four ranks of ingredients in the hierarchy of a prescription are the jun (usually translated into **monarch**, king, principal or chief), chen (usually translated into minister, **adjutant**, associate or deputy), zuo(usually translated into assistant or adjutant) and shi (usually translated into guide, messenger, conductant or **envoy**).

5   Not all prescriptions contain the full hierarchy of ingredients. In fact, it would be quite unusual for a prescription to include all the types of minister-ingredient, assistant-ingredient and guide-ingredient. Many prescriptions consist of only a monarch-ingredient and one or two minister-ingredients. If the monarch-ingredient and minister-ingredient are not toxic, there is no need for corrective assistant-ingredient. Sometimes the monarch-ingredient focuses on the location of the disorder, **obviating** the need for a guide-ingredient.

6   In practice, the hierarchy of ingredients is not always so clear-cut. While all prescriptions require a monarch-ingredient, sometimes the prescription is so well-balanced that it is difficult to distinguish the function served by each of its constituent ingredients. Examples are Wuwei Xiaodu Tang (*Five-Herb Decoction for Eliminating Toxin*) and Wupi San (*Five-Peel Powder*) in which all of the ingredients are accorded equal status. In other cases, the position of an ingredient in the hierarchy will vary depending on the particular circumstances for which the prescription is used. A typical example is Siwu Tang (*Four-Substance Decoction*) in which the relative **dosage** of the ingredients vary depending on whether its tonifying or invigorating

accentuate /əkˈsentʃueɪt/ *v*. 突出;强调

optimal /ˈɒptɪməl/ *adj*. 最佳的,最理想的
hierarchy /ˈhaɪərɑːkɪ/ *n*. 等级制度

monarch /ˈmɒnək/ *n*. 最高统治者;国王;女王;皇上;女皇
adjutant /ˈædʒutənt/ *n*. 副官;助手
envoy /ˈenvɔɪ/ *n*. 使者;代表;(尤指)外交官

obviate /ˈɒbvɪeɪt/ *v*. 排除;消除

dosage /ˈdəʊsɪdʒ/ *n*.(通常指药的)剂量

actions are emphasized.

7　In addition, for several of the prescriptions there has been intense debate over the centuries regarding which of the herbs is the monarch-ingredient. Such disagreement arises from different understandings of the **underlying** mechanism of the prescription, or even the condition for which the prescription is indicated. A typical example is Guizhi Shaoyao Zhimu Tang (*Ramulus Cinnamomi* , *Radix Paeoniae* and *Rhizoma Anemarrhenae Decoction*). There has been strong disagreement about whether the prescription is intended primarily for heat or cold disorders. As a result, Guizhi (*Ramulus Cinnamomi*), Mahuang (*Herba Ephedrae*), Baizhu (*Rhizoma Atractylodis Macrocephalae*), Zhimu (*Rhizoma Anemarrhenae*) and Fuzi (*Aconiti Praeparata*) has each been identified as the monarch-ingredient in the prescription.

8　The art of constructing a prescription requires more than a good grasp of the hierarchical principles discussed above. It also requires considerable flexibility in **tailoring** the prescription to fit the specific needs of the patient. Adjustments must be made for changes in the syndrome, the constitution of the patient, climate, and other environmental factors. This may involve altering the selection of herbs or their relative dosage, the method of preparation, or the means of administration. This ability to **modify** a prescription to fit a patient at a particular time is what distinguishes good practitioners from **mediocre** ones.

9　By modifying the dosage of ingredients, the strength of a prescription and even its indications may be altered. In some cases the modification may be significant enough to **warrant** consideration as a different prescription. Guizhi add Shaoyao Tang (*Ramulus Cinnamomi Decoction Plus Radix Paeoniae*) is an example of modifying the dosage of an herb to alter the **scope** of a prescription's indications. This prescription is identical to Guizhi Tang (*Ramulus Cinnamomi Decotion*) except that the dosage of Shaoyao (*Radix Paeoniae*) has been doubled. Because one of this herb's major actions is to alleviate abdominal pain, by doubling its dosage the modified prescription can be used in treating the same presentation for which this prescription is indicated, with the addition of abdominal fullness and pain.

10　The prescriptions are effective in treating disease **precisely** because of the nature and composition of their ingredients. When

underlie /ˌʌndəˈlaɪ/ *v.* 在(词等)下面划线；强化(态度、形势等)；加强；强调

tailor /ˈteɪlə/ *v.* 裁减

modify /ˈmɔdɪfaɪ/ *v.* 稍改；(尤指)使缓和，使改善；(在中医指)加减

mediocre /ˌmiːdɪˈəukə/ *n.* 不太好的；平庸的；二流的

warrant /ˈwɔrənt/ *vt.* 使有必要；使正当；使恰当

scope /skəup/ *n.* (处理、研究事物的)范围

precisely /prɪˈsaɪslɪ/ *adv.* 精确地；仔细地

one changes the ingredients, one changes the actions of the prescription. Generally, there are three types of ingredients modifications.

11   The first type occurs when the monarch-ingredient in the prescription and the main action of the prescription do not change, but minor ingredients are added or subtract ed to tune the prescription for a specific condition. For example, if a patient presents with symptoms for which *Ramulus Cinnamomi Decoction* is indicated, but also presents with wheezing, then Houpo (*Cortex Magnoliae Officinalis*) and Xingren (*Semen Pruni Armeniacae*) can be added. In this case, another prescription is created which is called Guizhi Houpo Xingren Tang (*Ramulus Cinnamomi Decoction plus Cortex Magnoliae Officinalis and Semen Pruni Armeniacae*).

12   In the second type of modification, the monarch-ingredient remains the same, but all or most of the other ingredients are changed so that the action of the prescription is also changed. Take for example the two-ingredient prescriptions in which Huanglian (*Rhizoma Coptidis*) is the monarch ingredient. If this herb is combined with Wuzhuyu (*Frucuts Evodiae*) acrid in taste and warm in nature which directs rebellious *qi* downward, the result is Zuojin Wan (*Left Metal Pill*). This prescription clears and drains fire from the liver, and thereby stops vomiting. It is used for constrained fire in the liver meridian with nausea, vomiting, hypochondriac pain and distension. On the other hand, if it is combined with Muxiang (*Radix Aucklandiae*) which promotes the movement of *qi*, the result is XianglianWan (*Aucklandia and Coptis Pill*). This prescription clears and dries damp-heat for dysenteric disorders due to damp-heat.

13   The third type of modification occurs when an alternation in the ingredients (sometimes only one ingredient) changes the prescription so fundamentally that its character, hierarchy, and actions are completely different. One of the best example is the transformation of Mahuang Tang (*Ephedra Decoction*), which is indicated for cold in the exterior, into Maxing Shigan Tang (*Ephedra, Semen Pruni Armeniacae, Gypsum Fibrosum and Radix Glycyrrhizae Decoction*), which is indicated for heat in the lungs. In this transformation, Shigao (*Gypsum Fibrosum*) is substituted for Guizhi (*Ramulus Cinnamomi*) as the minister-

subtract /səbˈtrækt/ *v.* 从（某数字）中减去（某数或量）

rebellious /rɪˈbeljəs/ *adj.* 叛逆的；难以控制的

constrain /kənˈstreɪn/ *v.* 限制；强迫

dysenteric /ˌdɪsənˈterɪk/ *adj.* 痢疾的

substitute /ˈsʌbstɪtjuːt/ *v.* 用某人或某物替代另外的人或物

ingredient.

14　Over the course of the past two thousand years medical practitioners in China have developed many different types of prescriptions to **administer** herbal medicine to their patients. Matching the appropriate type of **formulation** to the patient and disease is an important aspect of good practice. The development of new types of prescriptions has continued down to the present day. In fact it is here, perhaps more than in any other aspect of TCM, that modern technology is used on a wide scale. The commonly used types of prescriptions in TCM are Tang (decoctions), San (powders), Wan (pills), Gaoji (soft **extracts**), Danji (special pills), Tangjiangji (**syrup**), Jiuji (medicinal wines), Dingji (**lozenges**), Pianji (tablets), Chongfuji (**granules**) and Zhenji (injections). (1,325 words)

administer /əd'mɪnɪstə/ *v*. 正式发给或给予;(医学上指)给药

formulation /ˌfɔːmjuˈleɪʃən/ *n*. 格式化;公式化

extract /ɪkˈstrækt, ˈekstrækt/ *n*. 榨出物;浓缩物;(医学上)膏剂

syrup /ˈsɪrəp/ *n*. 糖浆;糖水;(医学上)糖浆剂

lozenge /ˈlɔzɪndʒ/ *n*. 糖锭;(尤指口含的)锭剂

granule /ˈɡrænjuːl/ *n*. 小颗粒;(医学上)冲服剂

Notes:

1. Like other aspects of traditional Chinese medicine, it is important to understand the nature of this development in order to clearly appreciate how the prescriptions came to be, and how to use them in the clinic to the best effect. 像中医的其他方面一样,了解方剂发展的本质对于理解方剂是如何形成的以及临床上如何应用才能取得最好的效果是很重要的。

2. They are complex recipes of interrelated substances, each of which affects the actions of the others in the prescription. 它们是由相关药物组成的复杂处方,方剂中的每一个成分都会影响其他成分的功效。

3. Every medicinal substance has its strengths and its shortcomings. 每一种药物都有其长处与不足。

4. An effective prescription is one in which the substances are carefully balanced to accentuate the strengths and reduce the side-effects. 一个有效的方剂,各成分之间的配伍要平衡以充分发挥其作用并减少副作用。

5. Constructing an effective prescription involves more than simply putting ingredients together to obtain a certain effect. 要组成一个方剂,简单地将各成分混合在一起并不就能获得一定的效果。

6. One needs an organizing principle to guide the construction so that the ingredients are combined in an optimal fashion. 需要知道一个组方的原则,这样各个成分才能以最佳的方式配伍在一起。

7. For this reason, the terms used to signify the importance or rank of the ingredients in a prescription reflect those used at court. 由于这个原因,表示各味药在一个方剂中的重要性或地位所使用的术语和宫廷的用语一样。

8. Sometimes the monarch-ingredient focuses on the level and location of the disorder, obviating the need for a guide-ingredient. 有时君药直接作用于患部及病位,这样就不需要使药了。

9. In practice, the hierarchy of ingredients is not always so clear-cut. 在实践中, 方剂中各味药的等级划分并不总是泾渭分明的。

10. In addition, for several of the prescriptions there has been intense debate over the centuries regarding which of the herbs is the monarch-ingredient. 另外, 有些方剂中到底何者为君药, 几百年来一直争论不休。

11. The art of constructing a prescription requires more than a good grasp of the hierarchical principles discussed above. 组方的方法并不局限于上面所讨论的等级原则。

12. It also requires considerable flexibility in tailoring the prescription to fit the specific needs of the patient. 拟定方剂以适应患者的特定需要, 这需要有相当的灵活性。

13. Adjustments must be made for changes in the syndrome, the strength of the patient, the season, climate, and other environmental factors. 组方时应根据病证、患者体质、季节、气候及其他环境因素作出相应的调整。

14. This may involve altering the selection of herbs or their relative dosage, the method of preparation, or the means of administration. 这可能涉及改变药物的选择或相关剂量、炮制的方法或给药的方式。

15. This ability to modify a prescription to fit a particular patient at a particular time is what distinguishes the very good practitioner from the mediocre. 加减处方以适应特定患者在特定时间治疗的能力是区分高明医家与庸医的标准。

16. The first type occurs when the monarch-ingredient in the prescription and the main action of the prescription do not change, but minor ingredients are added or subtracted to tune the prescription for a specific condition. 第一种方式, 君药和方剂的主要功效不变, 只是加上或去掉次要的成分以使方剂更适应于某一特定病证的治疗。

17. The third type of modification occurs when an alternation in the ingredients (sometimes only one ingredient) changes the prescription so fundamentally that its character, hierarchy, and actions are completely different. 第三种加减方式, 方中成分的改变导致了该方剂特点、等级排列和功效的彻底改变。

18. Matching the appropriate type of formulation to the patient and disease is an important aspect of good practice. 使组方适应于患者和疾病是治疗中非常重要的一环。

19. In fact it is here, perhaps more than in any other aspect to traditional Chinese medicine, that the influence of modern technology has been felt, as modern formulations and means of extraction are now used on a wide scale. 事实上, 正是在这里, 也许比中医其他领域都要突出, 现代技术的影响最为明显。因为现代组方技术和提取方法现在已得到了广泛的应用。

Task One　Reading Comprehension

1. According to the context, the phrase "came to be" (line 4, para. 1) may be best defined as _____ .

   A. came into being　　　　　　　B. worked together

   C. became effective　　　　　　　D. came from

2. In constructing an effective prescription, _____ is needed to guide the construction.

A. an orderly arrangement of ingredients

B. hierarchy of a prescription

C. an organizing principle

D. a rank of the ingredients

3. The advantage of a prescription and even its indications may have a big difference after _____ .

    A. selecting the herbs   B. discussing the hierarchical principles

    C. alleviating abdominal pain   D. modifying the dosage of ingredients

4. Three types of ingredients modifications mentioned in the text indicate _____ .

    A. prescriptions are constructed for a specific condition

    B. alternation of the ingredients will change the actions of the prescription

    C. prescription can be modified to fit a particular patient at a particular time

    D. fundamental changes of the prescription are completely different

5. According to the text, which of the following statement is **NOT** true?

    A. The hierarchy of ingredients is always easy to identify in practice.

    B. Every medicinal substance has its advantages and disadvantages.

    C. Not all prescriptions contain the full hierarchy of ingredients.

    D. Matching the appropriate type of formulation to the patient and disease is an important aspect of good practice.

Task Two　Vocabulary

1. Directions: Complete the following phrases respectively according to its corresponding meaning or equivalent in Chinese within the brackets.

1) in a _____ (累积的) fashion

2) complex _____ (相互作用)

3) _____ (突出) the strength

4) _____ (构建) an effective prescription

5) the four _____ (等级) of ingredients

6) _____ (矫正的) assistant-ingredient

7) _____ (组成的) ingredients

8) _____ (潜在的) mechanism

9) _____ (等级的) principles

10) considerable_____ (灵活性)

11) _____ (裁剪) the prescription

12) _____ (方法) of administration

13) distinguish good practitioners from _____ (平庸的) ones

14) _____ (使有必要) consideration

15) _____ (加倍) its dosage

16) _____ (次要的) ingredients

17) _____ （反抗的） *qi*

18) _____ （被约束的） fire

19) _____ （痢疾的） disorders

20) is _____ （替代的） for

2. Fill in the blanks with the words from the box and change the form when necessary.

hierarchy	monarch	accentuate	recipe	dosage
precisely	adjutant	modify	mediocre	warrant
subtract	constrain	rebellious	substitute	granule

1) Talley needed to _____ existing painkillers so that they attached only to enzymes with the protrusion.

2) Simvastatin （辛伐他丁） is currently marketed in _____ strengths of 5, 10, 20, 40, and 80 mg.

3) The _____ officers, having seized the radio station, broadcast the news of the overthrow （推翻） of the monarchy.

4) Microscopists （显微镜学家） can identify the source of starch （淀粉） by examination of _____ shape and arrangement.

5) It uses innovation training to create a new elite within its typically conservative social _____ .

6) His shaven head _____ his large round face.

7) The young teacher had to _____ for the sick colleague.

8) The real problem with drug prices is not so much that Sovaldi （一种治疗丙肝的药物） costs $84,000, but that so many _____ drugs cost about the same, or more.

9) The _____ of a country is the king, queen, emperor, or empress.

10) She learned household accounting — how to add and _____ bills for soap, candles, and flour.

11) But one ingredient never leaves the _____: their passion for making fresh delicious desserts.

12) The allegations （指控） are serious enough to _____ an investigation.

13) That has allowed General Wiranto, Mr Suharto's former _____ and now defense minister and commander-in-chief, to play a huge role in the negotiations.

14) It is _____ because the stakes are so high that a ceasefire has proved so elusive.

15) New York state, with more than 37,000 cases of the infectious disease, must be severely _____ for the moment.

Task Three   Writing

Please rewrite the text in a form of abstract （about 150 words）

Terminology

Basic Terminology of Chinese Materia Medica

Terminology	WHO	WFCMS
药	medicinal	medicinal; medicine
道地药材	authentic medicinal	genuine regional materia medica
炮制	processing of medicinals	processing of materia medica
切	cut the medicinal	cutting
水制	water processing	water processing
漂	long-rinse	rinsing
水飞	water-grind	grinding with water
火制	fire processing	fire processing
清炒	plain stir-bake	plain stir-frying
炒黄	stir-bake to yellow	stir-frying to yellow
炒焦	stir-bake to brown	stir-frying to brown
炒炭	stir-bake to scorch	stir-frying to scorch
炙	stir-bake with adjuvant	stir-frying with liquid adjuvant
煨	roast	roasting
烘焙	bake	baking
煅	calcine	calcining
中药性能	nature of medicinals	properties and actions of Chinese medicinal
升降浮沉	upbearing, downbearing, floating and sinking	ascending, descending, floating and sinking
归经	meridian entry	meridian/ channel tropism
配伍	combination	combination of medicinals
四气	four *qi*	four properties
去火毒	eliminate fire toxin	removing fire toxin
食忌	dietary contraindications	dietary contraindication
服药食忌	dietary contraindication during medication	dietary incompatibility
妊娠禁忌	contraindications during pregnancy	contraindication during pregnancy
十九畏	nineteen incompatibilities	nineteen mutual inhibitions
十八反	eighteen antagonisms	eighteen antagonisms
配伍禁忌	prohibited combination	prohibited combination
解表药	exterior-releasing medicinal	exterior-releasing medicinal

continued

Terminology	WHO	WFCMS
发散风寒药	wind-cold-dispersing medicinal	wind-cold-dispersing medicinal
辛温解表药	pungent-warm exterior-releasing medicinal	pungent-warm exterior-releasing medicinal
发散风热药	wind-heat-dispersing medicinal	wind-heat dispersing medicinal
辛凉解表药	pungent-cool exterior-releasing medicinal	pungent-cool exterior-releasing medicinal
清热药	heat-clearing medicinal	heat-clearing medicinal
清热泻火药	heat-clearing and fire-purging medicinal	heat-clearing and fire-purging medicinal
清热燥湿药	heat-clearing and dampness-drying medicinal	heat-clearing and dampness-drying medicinal
清热解毒药	heat-clearing and detoxicating medicinal	heat-clearing and detoxicating medicinal
清热凉血药	heat-clearing and blood-cooling medicinal	heat-clearing and blood-cooling medicinal
清虚热药	deficiency heat-clearing medicinal	deficiency-heat-clearing medicinal
泻下药	purgative medicinal	purgative medicinal
温下药	warm purgative medicinal	warm purgative
攻下药	offensive purgative medicinal	offensive purgative
润下药	laxative (medicinal)	laxative
峻下逐水药	drastic (purgative) water-expelling medicinal	drastic hydragogue
祛风湿药	wind-dampness-dispelling medicinal	wind-damp-dispelling medicinal
祛风湿散寒药	wind-dampness-dispelling and cold-dispersing medicinal	wind-damp-dispelling and cold-dissipating medicinal
祛风湿清热药	wind-dampness-dispelling and heat-clearing medicinal	wind-damp-dispelling and heat-clearing medicinal
化湿药	dampness-resolving medicinal	damp-resolving medicinal
利水渗湿药	dampness-draining diuretic medicinal	damp-draining diuretic
利水消肿药	water-draining and swelling-dispersing medicinal	edema-alleviating diuretic
利尿通淋药	strangury-relieving diuretic medicinal	stranguria-relieving diuretic
通淋药	strangury-relieving medicinal	stranguria-relieving medicinal
利湿退黄药	dampness-draining anti-icteric medicinal	damp-excreting anti-icteric medicinal
温里药	interior-warming medicinal	interior-warming medicinal
理气药	*qi*-regulating medicinal	*qi*-regulating medicinal
消食药	digestant medicinal	digestant medicinal
驱虫药	worm-expelling medicinal	vermifugal medicinal
止血药	hemostatic (medicinal)	hemostatic medicinal
凉血止血药	blood-cooling hemostatic medicinal	blood-cooling hemostatic
化瘀止血药	stasis-resolving hemostatic medicinal	stasis-resolving hemostatic
收敛止血药	astringent hemostatic medicinal	astringent hemostatic

continued

Terminology	WHO	WFCMS
温经止血药	meridian-warming hemostatic medicinal	meridian/channel-warming hemostatic
活血化瘀药	blood-activating and stasis-resolving medicinal	blood-activating and stasis-resolving medicinal
活血祛瘀药	blood-activating and stasis-dispelling medicinal	blood-activating and stasis-dispelling medicinal
活血行气药	blood-activating and *qi*-moving medicinal	blood-activating and *qi*-moving medicinal
活血止痛药	blood-activating analgesic medicinal	blood-activating analgesic
活血调经药	blood-activating menstruation-regulating medicinal	blood-activating and menstruation-regulating medicinal
活血疗伤药	blood-activating trauma-curing medicinal	blood-activating and trauma-curing medicinal
破血消癥药	blood-breaking mass-eliminating medicinal	medicinal for breaking blood stasis and eliminating mass
止咳平喘药	cough-suppressing and panting-calming medicinal	antitussive and antiasthmatic medicinal
安神药	tranquilizing medicinal	tranquilizer; tranquilizing medicinal
重镇安神药	settling tranquilizing medicinal	settling tranquilizer
养心安神药	heart-nourishing tranquillizing medicinal	heart-nourishing tranquillizer
平肝息风药	liver-pacifying and wind-extinguishing medicinal	liver-pacifying wind-extinguishing medicinal
开窍药	orifice-opening medicinal	resuscitative stimulant; resuscitative medicinal
补益药	tonifying and replenishing medicinal	tonic; tonifying medicinal
补气药	*qi*-tonifying medicinal	*qi* tonic; *qi*-tonifying medicinal
补血药	blood-tonifying medicinal	blood tonic; blood-tonifying medicinal
养血药	blood-tonifying medicinal	blood-tonifying medicinal
柔肝药	liver-emolliating medicinal	liver-emolliating medicinal
补阳药	*yang*-tonifying medicinal	*yang* tonic; *yang*-tonifying medicinal
补肾阳药	kidney *yang*-tonifying medicinal	kidney-*yang* tonic; kidney *yang*-tonifying medicinal
补阴药	*yin*-tonifying medicinal	*yin* tonic; *yin*-tonifying medicinal
收涩药	astringent medicinal	astringent medicinal
固涩药	astringent medicinal	astringent medicinal
固表止汗药	exterior-securing anhidrotic medicinal	exterior-strengthening anhidrotic medicinal
敛汗固表药	sweat-constraining exterior-securing medicinal	sweat-arresting and exterior-strengthening medicinal
敛肺涩肠药	lung-intestine astringent medicinal	lung-intestine astringent medicinal
涌吐药	emetic medicinal	emetic medicinal
方剂	formula	formula
经方	classical formula	classical formula

continued

Terminology	WHO	WFCMS
理法方药	principles, methods, formulas and medicinals	principle-method-recipe-medicinal
大方	major formula	large formula
小方	minor formula	minor formula
缓方	slow-acting formula	mild formula
急方	quick-acting formula	emergent formula
奇方	odd-numbered formula	odd-ingredient formula
偶方	even-numbered formula	even-ingredient formula
复方	compound formula	compound formula
八阵	eight tactical arrays	eight tactical arrays
君臣佐使	sovereign, minister, assistant and courier	sovereign, minister, assistant and guide
君药	sovereign medicinal	sovereign medicinal
臣药	minister medicinal	minister medicinal
佐药	assistant medicinal	assistant medicinal
使药	courier medicinal	guiding medicinal
反佐	counteracting assistant	using corrigent
剂型	preparation form	dosage form
汤剂	decoction (preparation)	decoction
片剂	tablet (preparation)	tablet
条剂	medicinal strip	medicated roll
膏剂	paste preparation	paste
散剂	powder preparation	powder
丸剂	pill preparation	pill
颗粒剂	soluble granules	granule
冲剂	soluble granules	infusion granule
茶剂	medicated tea	medicated tea
针剂	injection	injection
栓剂	suppository	suppository
丹剂	pellet	pellet
酒剂	medicated wine	wine preparation
膏药	plaster	plaster
浸膏	extract	extract
软膏	ointment	ointment; unguentum
蜡丸	waxed pill	wax pill
糊丸	pasted pill	flour and water paste pill

continued

Terminology	WHO	WFCMS
蜜丸	honeyed pill	honeyed pill
药线	medicated thread	medicated thread
煎药法	decoction method	decocting method
水煎	decoct with water	decocted with water
先煎	decoct first	to be decocted first
后下	decoct later	to be decocted later
包煎	wrap-decoct	wrap-boiling
另煎	decoct separately	decocted separately
单煎	decoct separately	decocted alone
溶化	dissolve	dissolve
冲服	take drenched	take infused
顿服	take in one single dose	administered at draught
代茶服(饮)	take as tea	taking as tea
临睡服	take before sleeping	administered before sleeping
平旦服	take before breakfast	administrated before breakfast
文火	slow fire	mild fire
武火	strong fire	strong fire
发表剂	exterior-effusing formula	exterior-relieving formula
清热剂	heat-clearing formula	heat-clearing formula
泻火剂	fire-draining/reducing formula	fire-purging formula
清暑剂	summerheat-clearing formula	summerheat-clearing formula
祛暑剂	summerheat-clearing formula	summerheat-dispelling formula
攻下剂	purgative formula	offensive purgative formula
攻里剂	interior-attacking formula	interior-attacking formula
寒下剂	cold purgative formula	cold purgative formula
润下剂	lubricant laxative formula	lubricant laxative formula
和解剂	harmonizing and releasing formula	harmonizing formula
表里双解剂	exterior-interior-releasing formula	exterior-interior dual releasing formula
温里剂	cold-dispelling formula	warming interior formula
祛寒剂	cold-dispelling formula	cold-dispelling formula
固涩剂	securing and astringent formula	astringent formula
理血剂	blood-regulating formula	blood-regulating formula
治风剂	wind-dispelling formula	wind-relieving formula
祛风剂	wind-dispelling formula	wind-dispelling formula

continued

Terminology	WHO	WFCMS
治燥剂	dryness-treating formula	dryness-relieving formula
润燥剂	dryness-moistening formula	dryness-moistening formula
祛湿剂	dampness-dispelling formula	dampness-dispelling formula
祛痰剂	phlegm-dispelling formula	phlegm-expelling formula
除痰剂	phlegm-dispelling formula	phlegm-eliminating formula
消食剂	digestant formula	digestive formula
消导剂	digestant formula	digestive and evacuative formula
驱虫剂	worm-expelling formula	anthelmintic formula
经产剂	formula for menstruation and childbirth	formula for menstruation and childbirth
痈疡剂	formula for treating abscess and ulcer	formula for treating abscess and ulcer
明目剂	vision-improving formula	vision-improving formula
救急剂	emergency formula	emergency formula

本书配套数字教学资源

微信扫描二维码，加入中医英语
读者交流圈，获取配套教学视
频、学习课件、课后习题和沟通交
流平台等板块内容，夯实基础知识

Those who are good at acupuncture treat diseases just like
removing thorns, cleaning contamination,
undoing knots and dredging stagnation.
夫善用针者,取其疾也,犹拔刺也,
犹雪污也,犹解结也,犹决闭也①。

Unit 9 Introduction to Acupuncture and Moxibustion

Warming-up

Before you listen (Watch)

In this section you will watch a video clip about "Acupuncture and moxibustion of TCM". The following words and phrases may be of help.

insertion /ɪnˈsɜːrʃn/	n.	插入
moxa /ˈmɒksə/	n.	艾;灸料
stem from	v.	起源于
stability /stəˈbɪlətɪ/	n.	稳定
upset /ʌpˈset/	a.	混乱的
puncture /ˈpʌŋktʃər/	v.	刺穿
Artemisia /ˌɑrtɪˈmɪzɪə/	n.	艾;艾属
dredge /dredʒ/	v.	疏浚
twirl /twɜːrl/	v.	转动
grind /graɪnd/	v.	研磨

While you listen(Watch)

Listen to the passage carefully and fill in each of the blanks marked from 1) to 10) according to what you have heard.

The techniques of acupuncture and moxibustion in traditional Chinese medicine are a

---

① 《灵枢·九针十二原》,李照国译。

traditional knowledge and practice formed in the soil of ancient Chinese culture for regulating the body's balance and 1) _____ health. They're based on the holistic concept of unity between man and nature. Under the guidance of the theories of the channels and acupuncture points, its practice involves the 2) _____ of needles into specific points on the body or the burning of moxa to warm the surface parts of the body in order to relieve pain, treat illness, or promote health.

The holistic concept of unity between man and nature, which stems from ancient Chinese philosophy, views the living individual a 3) _____ part of the universe and explains life activities with the theory of *yin* and *yang*.

For instance, in the natural world, *yin* represents the earth, the moon and night, whereas *yang* represents the sky or heaven, the sun and day. Inside the human body upward movement represents *yang*, where 4) _____ and downward movement represents *yin*.

Yin and *yang* govern nature as well as the body's interior. Therefore, if the *yin*-*yang* balance between the 5) _____ environment and the body or that within the body is 6) _____, disease results.

The theories of acupuncture and moxibustion hold the human body is a 7) _____, each part of which is connected by channels. Through long term practice, points on the channels have been discovered, gradually developing into a 8) _____ theory of which the 12 channels correspond to the 12 months and 365 acupuncture points to the 365 days of the year. This theory embodies the 9) _____ relationship between heaven, man and earth. For instance, if a patient has a toothache on the left side, it can be treated by inserting a needle in the *hegu* point on the right hand.

The principle of selecting points on the lower body for diseases in the upper, or of selecting points on the right for diseases on the left reflects clearly acupuncture and moxibustion's holistic view of the human body as an 10) _____ whole.

After you listen(Watch)

Please discuss with your partner the following questions and give your presentation to the class.

1) What is the practice of acupuncture and moxibustion like?

2) How do you understand "the human body is a microcosm"?

3) How are moxa cones and sticks made?

4) What are the health benefits of acupuncture and moxibustion?

Reading

 Text A

BEFORE CLASS

1. Quest for Definition

Directions: Explore online the definitions of the following terms from Text A and prepare a unique *one-minute* oral presentation for your class.

1) meridians and collaterals

2) acupoints

3) meridian acupoints

4) extraordinary acupoints

5) Ashi acupoints

6) special acupoints

2. Text-based Activities

Directions: Read carefully the part of Text A that corresponds to your task, and then prepare a unique *one-minute* oral presentation for your class.

PERFORMANCE IN CLASS

Your Task

1) What is the purpose of stimulating certain acupoints in the application of acupuncture and moxibustion?

2) What functions of acupuncture and moxibustion have been proved by experiments?

3) How can acupoints be classified? What are they respectively?

4) Briefly introduce ten types of special acupoints in our body and their efficacy in clinical treatment.

5) What are the requirements involved in the therapy of acupuncture and moxibustion?

Acupuncture and Moxibustion

1   Acupuncture and moxibustion are important component procedures in TCM which prevent and treat diseases by means of needling certain **acupoints** located on the body with **metallic** needles① or

---

①   metallic needles: 金属针。

stimulating certain regions on the body by applying heat with **ignited** moxa wool①. Since they are highly effective, simple in performance and low in cost, they have been widely used in China and neighboring countries for thousands of years.

2   The application of acupuncture and moxibustion through stimulating certain acupoints on the human body is to activate the meridians and collaterals and to regulate the function of the internal organs, qi and blood so as to prevent and treat diseases.

3   Experiments have proved that acupuncture and moxibustion can strengthen the central nervous system and especially reinforce the action of the **sympathetic** nervous system② and **cerebral cortex** ③ which control all the **tissues** and organs of the human body. For instance, acupuncture and moxibustion can regulate heartbeat, body temperature, blood pressure and respiration; relieve muscle **spasm** and numbness; treat disorders of **exocrine** and **endocrinesecretions**; and promote secretion of the **glands**, such as **pituitary**, **thyroid**, **parathyroid**, **adrenic**, sweat, **pancreatic** and digestive glands.

4   The treatment of acupuncture and moxibustion is based on acupoints. Acupoints are the regions where *qi* and blood from the viscera and meridians **effuse** and **infuse** beneath the body surface, usually located in the interstices of the thick muscles or between tendons and bones④. Acupoints generally can be classified into three categories, i. e, meridian acupoints, extraordinary acupoints and Ashi acupoints⑤.

5   Meridian acupoints, also known as acupoints of the fourteen meridians, refer to the acupoints located on the twelve meridians as well as the governor and conception vessels⑥. Meridian acupoints, the main part of the acupoints and frequently selected for acupuncture treatment, pertain to definite meridians with fixed names and locations⑦.

6   Extraordinary acupoints refer to the acupoints excluding the ones located on the fourteen meridians. These acupoints have definite locations and names and are effective in treating certain diseases. But they usually do not **pertain** to any meridians. However, the extraordinary acupoints and meridian acupoints are closely related to each other. Some extraordinary acupoints include certain meridian acupoints.

7   Ashi acupoints actually refer to **tenderness**⑧. Such acupoints are characterized by absence of fixed locations, definite names and pertaining meridians.

8   In acupuncture and moxibustion, there are still some specific acupoints that are located on the

---

①   ignited moxa wool：燃烧着的艾绒。

②   sympathetic nervous system：交感神经系统。

③   cerebral cortex：大脑皮质。

④   tendons and bones：筋骨。

⑤   Acupoints generally can be classified into three categories, i. e, meridian acupoints, extraordinary acupoints and Ashi acupoints：腧穴一般可以分为三类：即经穴、奇穴和阿是穴。

⑥   governor and conception vessels：任督二脉。

⑦   pertain to definite meridians with fixed names and locations：归属于一定的经脉并有固定的名称和定位。

⑧   Ashi acupoints actually refer to tenderness：阿是穴实际上指的是压痛点。

fourteen meridians with special curative effects. A majority of these acupoints are commonly used in clinical treatment.

9   There are ten types of special acupoints including five Shu acupoint①, *Yuan-Source* acupoints②, *Luo-Connective* acupoint③, Lower *He-Sea* acupoints④, *Xi-Cleft* acupoints⑤ and eight **convergence** acupoints⑥ below the knees and elbows; *Back-Shu* acupoints⑦ and *Front-Mu* acupoints⑧ located on the trunk; as well as eight **confluent** acupoints⑨ and crossing acupoints⑩ located on the whole body.

10   The five Shu acupoints — *Jing-Well*, *Ying-Spring*, *Shu-Stream*, *Jing-River* and *He-Sea* — are located on the twelve meridians below the knees and elbows or knees⑪. They are situated in the above mentioned order from the distal **extremities** ⑫ to the elbows or knees. From these five acupoints, we can see the indication of acupoints below the knees and elbows.

11   The Yuan-Source acupoints, as the regions where the primary qi of the viscera flows through and retains, are usually located around the wrists and ankles⑬. Those points can reflect the pathological changes of the viscera. Therefore, they are clinically used to diagnose and treat the disorders of the related viscera.

12   The Luo-Connecting acupoints refer to the acupoints from which the fifteen collaterals stem from the twelve meridians, the governor and conception vessels as well as the major collateral of the spleen⑭. All the Luo-Connecting acupoints of the twelve meridians are located below the elbows and knees. These acupoints are used to treat disorders of the regions that the meridians and collaterals run through as well as to those that the meridians are externally and internally related to each other.

---

①   five Shu acupoint：五腧穴。
②   *Yuan-Source* acupoints：原穴。
③   *Luo-Connective* acupoint：络穴。
④   Lower *He-Sea* acupoints：下合穴。
⑤   *Xi-Cleft* acupoints：郄穴。
⑥   eight convergence acupoints：八会穴。
⑦   *Back-Shu* acupoints：背俞穴。
⑧   *Front-Mu* acupoints：募穴。
⑨   eight confluent acupoints：八脉交会穴。
⑩   crossing acupoints：交会穴。
⑪   The five Shu acupoints — *Jing-Well*, *Ying-Spring*, *Shu-Stream*, *Jing-River* and *He-Sea* — are located on the twelve meridians below the knees and elbows or knees：五腧穴指十二经脉分布在肘、膝关节以下的五个特定穴位，分别名为井、荥、输、经、合穴。
⑫   distal extremities：四肢末端。
⑬   The Yuan-Source acupoints, as the regions where the primary qi of the viscera flows through and retains, are usually located around the wrists and ankles：原穴通常分布于腕、踝关节附近，是脏腑原气输注、经过和留止的部位。
⑭   The Luo-Connecting acupoints refer to the acupoints from which the fifteen collaterals stem from the twelve meridians, the governor and conception vessels as well as the major collateral of the spleen：络穴指位于络脉从十二经脉、任督二脉以及脾之大络别出部位的穴位。

13   The *Xi-Cleft* acupoints are the sites where *qi* and blood from the meridians are deeply converged①. Each of the twelve meridians and the four extraordinary meridians has a *Xi-Cleft* acupoint on the limbs, amounting to sixteen in all. All the *Xi-cleft* acupoints, except Liangqiu (ST 34)② on the stomach meridian, are all situated below the knees and elbows. Clinically, *Xi-Cleft* acupoints are used to treat severe acute disorders of meridians. The *Xi-Cleft* acupoints on the *yin* meridians are usually used to treat various blood syndromes and the *Xi-Cleft* acupoints on the *yang* meridians are often used to treat various pain syndromes.

14   The eight confluent acupoints refer to the eight acupoints on the twelve meridians that are connected with the eight extraordinary meridians③. These eight acupoints are all located below the knees and elbows and are used to treat disorders involving the face, head and trunk related to the eight extraordinary meridians.

15   The lower *He-Sea* acupoints refer to the six acupoints located on the three *yang* meridians of the foot where *qi* from the six *fu*-organs converge. They are the key acupoints for treating the disorders of the six *fu*-organs④.

16   The *Back-Shu* acupoints are located on the back and waist along the first lateral line of the bladder meridian (1. 5 *cun* lateral to the back midline). And they are the regions where *qi* of the viscera is infused⑤. The distributing order of *Back-Shu* acupoints is similar to that of the location of the *zang*-organs and *fu*-organs. Clinically, these acupoints are used to treat the disorders of the related viscera, tissues and organs.

17   The Front-Mu acupoints are those located on the chest and abdomen where *qi* of the viscera infuses and converges⑥. The location of the *Front-Mu* acupoints is similar to that of the related *zang*-organs and *fu*-organs. Among these acupoints, six on the conception vessel are **unilateral** acupoints and the rest are **bilateral** ones. *Front-Mu* acupoints can be used to treat disorders of the related viscera, especially the disorder of six *fu*-organs. These acupoints are usually needled with the combination of *Back-Shu* acupoints.

---

①   The *Xi-Cleft* acupoints are the sites where qi and blood from the meridians are deeply converged：郄穴是各经经气所深聚的地方。

②   Liangqiu (ST34)：梁丘 Liángqiū (ST34)。在股前外侧,髌底上 2 寸,股外侧肌与股直肌肌腱之间。穴位命名采用 1991 年世界卫生组织总部颁布的国际标准《国际针灸命名推荐标准》(*A proposed Standard International Acupuncture Nomenclature*)。根据该标准,针灸穴名包括三个要素：汉字、汉语拼音和国际代码。

③   The eight confluent acupoints refer to the eight acupoints on the twelve meridians that are connected with the eight extraordinary meridians：八脉交会穴指奇经八脉与十二正经脉气相通的八个腧穴。

④   The lower *He-Sea* acupoints refer to the six acupoints located on the three yang meridians of the foot where qi from the six *fu*-organs converge. They are the key acupoints for treating the disorders of the six *fu*-organs：下合穴是六腑之气下合于下肢足三阳经的六个腧穴,是治疗六腑证的要穴。

⑤   The *Back-Shu* acupoints are located on the back and waist along the first lateral line of the bladder meridian (1.5 *cun* lateral to the back midline). And they are the regions where qi of the viscera is infused：背俞穴位于背腰部足太阳膀胱经的第一侧线上(后正中线旁开 1.5 寸),是脏腑之气输注之处。

⑥   The *Front-Mu* acupoints are those located on the chest and abdomen where qi of the viscera infuses and converges：募穴位于胸腹部,是脏腑之气汇聚之处。

18　The eight influential acupoints, located on the trunk and four limbs, are the regions where essence of *qi*, blood, tendons, vessels, bones, marrow, *zang*-organs and *fu*-organs converge①.

19　The crossing acupoints are those located at the **intersections** of two or more meridian②. Most of them are located on the head, face and trunk, the rest are located on the lower limbs. The crossing acupoints state the fact that indication of acupoints is composed of two parts, namely the four limbs and regions on the head and trunk. Clinically, these acupoints are used to treat disorders of the crossing meridians.

20　There are various methods for the manipulation of acupuncture and moxibustion. The action of these manipulating techniques is generally summarized as being either reinforcing or reducing③. The former means to strengthen body resistance while the latter means to eliminate pathogenic factors. The therapy of acupuncture and moxibustion also involves various requirements such as accurate location of the acupoints, proper **insertion** of the needle, necessary retention of the needle and correct withdrawal of the needle.

New Words and Expressions

acupoint /ˈækjʊpɒɪnt/ *n*. any of the specific points on the body where a needle is inserted in acupuncture or pressure is applied in acupressure 穴位

metallic /məˈtælɪk/ *adj*. made of metal or containing metal 金属的

ignite /ɪɡˈnaɪt/ *v*. to start burning, or to make something start burning 燃烧；点火

sympathetic /ˌsɪmpəˈθetɪk/ *adj*. of or relating to the division of the autonomic-nervous system that acts in opposition to the parasympathetic system accelerating the heartbeat, dilating the bronchi, inhibiting the smooth muscles of the digestive tract, etc 交感神经的

reinforce /ˌriːɪnˈfɔːs/ *v*. make sth. stronger by adding material, etc; emphasize 增强，加强

cerebral /səˈriːbrəl/ *adj*. of the brain 大脑的；脑的

cortex /ˈkɔːteks/ *n*. outer layer of the brain or other organ（脑或其他器官的）皮

tissue /ˈtɪʃuː/ *n*. mass of cells forming the body of an animal or a plant 组织

spasm /ˈspæzəm/ *n*. a painful and involuntary muscular contraction 痉挛

exocrine /ˈeksəʊkraɪn/ *adj*. of or relating to exocrine glands or their secretions 外分泌的

endocrine /ˈendəʊkraɪn/ *adj*. of or belonging to endocrine glands or their secretions 内分泌的

secretion /sɪˈkriːʃn/ *n*. a substance, usually liquid, produced by part of a plant or animal 分泌物

gland /ɡlænd/ *n*. any of various organs that synthesize substances needed by the body and release it through ducts or directly into the bloodstream 腺

---

①　The eight influential acupoints, located on the trunk and four limbs, are the regions where essence of *qi*, blood, tendons, vessels, bones, marrow, *zang*- organs and *fu*-organs converge：八会穴分散于躯干部和四肢部，是脏、腑、气、血、筋、脉、骨、髓等精气所会聚的腧穴。

②　The crossing acupoints are those located at the intersections of two or more meridian：交会穴是两经或数经相交会的腧穴。

③　The action of these manipulating techniques is generally summarized as being either reinforcing or reducing：这些针刺手法的功效可以概括为补或泻。

pituitary /pɪˈtjuːɪtərɪ/ *adj.* of or relating to the pituitary gland 垂体的

thyroid /ˈθaɪrɔɪd/ *adj.* of or relating to the thyroid gland 甲状腺的

parathyroid /ˌpærəˈθaɪrɔɪd/ *adj.* of or relating to the parathyroid gland 甲状旁腺的

adrenic /əˈdrenɪk/ *adj.* of or relating to the adrenal gland 肾上腺的

pancreatic /ˌpæŋkrɪˈætɪk/ *adj.* of or relating to the pancreas 胰腺的

effuse /ɪˈfjuːz/ *v.* pour or flow out, especially of liquid 流出；倾出

infuse /ɪnˈfjuːz/ *v.* fill, as with a certain quality 注入

pertain /pəˈteɪn/ *v.* be relevant to 与……相关

tenderness /ˈtendənəs/ *n.* a pain that is felt when the area is touched 压痛点

convergence /kənˈvɜːdʒəns/ *n.* the occurrence of two or more things coming together 汇于一点；聚集

confluent /ˈkɒnfluənt/ *adj.* flowing or coming together; uniting 汇合的

extremity /ɪkˈstremətɪ/ *n.* one of the parts of your body that is furthest away from the centre, for example your fingers and toes 肢

unilateral /ˌjuːnɪˈlætrəl/ *adj.* involving only one part or side 单方向的，单侧的

bilateral /ˌbaɪˈlætərəl/ *adj.* involving two parties or sides 双侧的

intersection /ˌɪntəˈsekʃn/ *n.* a point at which things intersect 交点，交叉

FOLLOW-UP ACTIVITIES

Task one   Comprehension Check

1. Questions for Discussion

1) On what basis are acupoints chosen in clinical therapy?

2) Do you know why Ashi acupoint was so named?

3) Why is acupuncture and moxibustion usually used together literally?

4) What are the differences between the heat-sensitive moxibustion and the traditional moxibustion?

2. Chart completion

INTRODUCTION: (para. 1 - 3)
　　Acupuncture and moxibustion can prevent and treat diseases through 1) ＿＿＿＿＿＿
＿＿＿＿＿＿＿ in order to 2) ＿＿＿＿＿＿＿＿＿ and 3) ＿＿＿＿＿＿＿＿＿ .

THE CLASSIFICATION OF ACUPOINTS: (para. 4 - 19)
- Acupoints can be classified into three categories: meridian acupoints, 4) ＿＿＿＿＿＿
＿＿＿＿＿＿＿ .
- There are ten types of special acupoints located on the 14 meridians, they are 5) ＿＿＿＿
＿＿＿＿＿＿＿＿＿＿＿＿＿＿＿＿＿＿＿＿＿＿＿＿＿＿＿＿＿＿＿＿＿＿＿＿＿
＿＿＿＿＿＿＿＿＿＿＿＿＿＿＿＿＿＿＿＿ .

THE PRACTICE OF ACUPUNCTURE AND MOXIBUSTION：（para. 20）

The action of manipulating acupuncture and moxibustion can be summarized as 6) _____ _____ . To ensure the effectiveness of acupuncture and moxibustion, the following 4 aspects should be taken into consideration, they are：the accurate location of the acupoints, 7) _____ , 8) _____ , and 9) _____ _____ .

Task Two　Vocabulary

1. Directions：Complete the following phrases respectively according to its corresponding meaning or equivalent in Chinese within the brackets.

1) _____（燃烧的）moxa wool

2) activate the meridians and _____（络）

3) _____（刺激）certain acupoints

4) all _____（组织）and organs

5) relieve muscle _____（痉挛）

6)（内分泌的）_____ secretions

7) _____（经络）

8) _____（加强）the central nervous system

9) ashi acupoints refer to_____（痛点）

10) _____（调节）heartbeat

11) the _____（缝隙）of thick muscles

12) _____（和……相关）to any meridians

13) distal _____（肢）

14) _____（严重急性的）disorders

15) _____（单侧的）acupoints

16) _____（操作）of acupuncture and moxibustion

17) _____（补）or reduce

18) proper _____（插入）of the needle

19) the _____（疗法）of acupuncture and moxibustion

20) _____（金属的）needle

21) _____（筋）and bones

22) _____（任督）vessels

23) to _____（消除）pathogenic factors

24) _____（原气）of the viscera

25) various _____（血证）

26) be _____（分类）into three categories

27) _____（停留）of the needle

28) _____（of foot *taiyang*）（足太阳膀胱经）

29) _____（交点）of two or more meridians

30) strengthen body_____（抵抗力）

2. Match the following words with their proper meanings.

Column I	Column II
1) activate	a. the power to produce an effect
2) application	b. to make active or more active
3) clinical	c. to recognize (something, such as a disease) by signs and symptoms
4) internal	d. partial or total lack of sensation in a part of the body; a symptom of nerve damage or dysfunction
5) efficacy	e. of, relating to, or occurring on the inside of an organized structure (such as a club, company, or state)
6) diagnose	f. an act of putting something to use
7) relieve	g. to bring about the removal or alleviation of
8) influential	h. a group of signs and symptoms that occur together and characterize a particular abnormality or condition
9) numbness	i. of, relating to, or conducted in or as if in a clinic, such as involving direct observation of the patient
10) syndrome	j. having or exercising influence or power
11) manipulation	k. a retraction of a previously held position or the act of withdrawing
12) eliminate	l. to divide them into groups or types so that things with similar characteristics are in the same group
13) retention	m. terminate, end, or take out
14) withdrawal	n. the act of retaining
15) classify	o. skillful management or utilization

3. Fill in the blanks with the words from the box and change the form when necessary.

clinical	activate	withdrawal	syndrome	bilateral
sympathetic	manipulation	convergence	tissue	classify
numbness	intersection	efficacy	pertain	internal

1) Some healthcare providers are _____ to the hospital administrators, who are dealing with a lack of critical resources during an unprecedented pandemic.

2) When not working on creative projects, Wendy also provides nutritional counseling and diabetes management to clients in a _____ setting.

3) It used a flashlight-like device to _____ photo cells on the television set to change channels.

4) The meeting came as Iraq's government seemed to embrace parts of Obama's plan for

_____ of U.S. troops.

5) The extent to which liquid biopsy (活组织检查) might ultimately replace standard _____ biopsies is still unclear.

6) But with that longer life, people with Downs (唐氏) _____ may have an increased risk for Alzheimer's (老年痴呆症) disease at an early age.

7) Of course in the reversible case, you're always pushing against an external pressure, which is essentially equal to the _____ pressure.

8) Obviously not everything that improves your health comes in a pill bottle, but there are strict standards used by the FDA to prove safety and _____ before things like a drug or medical device goes to market.

9) Meanwhile, frozen skiers and snowboarders disembark from the lift complaining about _____ fingers and toes.

10) More information _____ to the case was expected to be discussed at a press briefing scheduled for later on Tuesday.

11) Economists and government officials have rejected the idea that Brazil and Argentina are intentionally _____ their currencies (货币).

12) Vaccines that contain a living, weakened pathogen — such as the vaccines against measles and tuberculosis — _____ the immune system generally, Aaby and Stabell Benn say, making recipients better able to fight off other infections.

13) However, Ardern was criticized this week for failing to raise the topic of climate change in her first _____ meeting with Donald Trump.

14) After the Second World War, mathematics in the United States flourished owing to a _____ of interests.

15) This article is part of our latest Museums special section, which focuses on the _____ of art and politics.

Task Three   Translation
1   Translate the following medical expressions into English.

1) 阿是穴   2) 五腧穴
3) 原穴   4) 增强中枢神经系统
5) 络穴   6) 奇穴
7) 下合穴   8) 募穴
9) 八会穴   10) 八脉交会穴
11) 治疗内分泌失调   12) 痛证
13) 拔针   14) 双穴
15) 背俞穴   16) 消除致病因素
17) 郄穴   18) 交会穴
19) 促进腺体分泌   20) 胃经

2　Translate the following sentences into Chinese or English.

1. Since acupuncture and moxibustion are highly effective, simple in performance and low in cost, they have been widely used in China and neighboring countries for thousands of years.

2. Extraordinary acupoints refer to the acupoints excluding the ones located on the fourteen meridians. These acupoints have definite locations and names and are effective in treating certain diseases.

3. Acupoints are the regions where *qi* and blood from the viscera and meridians effuse and infuse beneath the body surface, usually located in the interstices of the thick muscles or between tendons and bones.

4. The *Xi-Cleft* acupoints on the *yin* meridians are usually used to treat various blood syndromes and the *Xi-Cleft* acupoints on the *yang* meridians are often used to treat various pain syndromes.

5. The therapy of acupuncture and moxibustion also involves various requirements such as accurate location of the acupoints, proper insertion of the needle, necessary retention of the needle and correct withdrawal of the needle.

6. 常用的进针手法主要分为单手进针法和双手进针法。(be classified into)

7. 阿是穴的特征是既无具体的名称，也无特定的位置。(be characterized by)

8. 经穴主要指分布于十二经脉和任督二脉上的腧穴。(refer to, located)

9. 针灸减肥主要是通过调整机体的代谢功能，促进脂肪分解，达到减肥减脂的效果。(by means of)

10. 临床试验证明热敏灸大幅度提高了艾灸治疗难治病症的疗效。(prove, efficacy)

3　Translate the following passage into English.

热敏灸是采用点燃的艾材产生的艾热悬灸热敏态穴位，激发透热、扩热、传热、局部不(微)热远部热、表面不(微)热深部热、非热觉等热敏灸感和经气传导，并施以个体化的饱和消敏灸量，从而提高艾灸疗效的一种新疗法，在当前针灸界有重要影响。

◥ Text B

Moxibustion

1　Moxibustion uses **moxa**, or its products, to **blister** the skin or to make the skin warm. Moxa is in season from March to May. After picking the leaves, put them in a cool shade to dry, then place them in a stone bowl and crush them until they **crumble**. Then put the moxa through a **sieve**, **sifting** away dirt, rocks, etc. The moxa is ready to use when it is clean, thin and soft.

2　There are many methods of using moxibustion, but the most common is burning a piece of moxa on or near the skin. This

moxa /ˈmɒksə/ *n.* 艾绒

blister /ˈblɪstə(r)/ *v.* (使)起疱, 起泡

crumble /ˈkrʌmbl/ *v.* (使)破碎, 成碎屑

sieve /sɪv/ *n.* 滤器; 筛子; 筷篱; 漏勺

sift /sɪft/ *v.* 筛(面粉或颗粒

method is called moxa-**cone** method which is either direct or indirect. This method uses small pyramid-shaped piles of moxa known as Zhu (cone) in Chinese. A cone after it has been burned is called one Zhuang, that means the burning of one moxa cone. The size of the moxa cone and the number of applications that must be used will differ, depending on the severity of disease. For a person who is comparatively healthy and is in the beginning stage of a disease, one should use a large moxa cone, and many applications, whereas a person who is less healthy and has a chronic illness should be treated with small cones and fewer applications. When using moxa on the head, face, fingers and chest area, the moxa cones should be small and the applications few. When treating the back and stomach area, larger cones and more applications can be used.

3   The rule of thumb is: On fleshy areas, bigger cones and more applications can be used, whereas on less fleshy parts of the body, the cones should be small and the applications few. One should also use less moxa and fewer applications on children and old patients. For patients with serious illnesses, where much moxa should be applied many times, but whose health or age prevents this, smaller cones should be used but the applications increased.

4   The size of the moxa cone differs in the moxa-cone method. Less moxa should be used in the direct method than in the indirect one. In making moxa cone, one can use hands to roll the moxa into a pyramid shape. A big cone is about the size of a **Lima bean** (1 cm tall, 0.8 cm in diameter and 0.1 gm in weight) and is used in the indirect method. The middle-sized cone is about the size of a soybean, while the small cone is about the size of a grain of wheat.

5   The direct method of moxibustion can be divided into two categories: the blister-producing method, and the non-blister-producing method. As their names imply, the blister-producing method will burn the skin and produce a blister, while the non-blister-producing method will not.

6   The indirect method, unlike the direct method, does not burn the moxa directly on the skin. Instead, it uses some kind of middle layer. The three most common indirect methods are: the ginger method, the garlic method, and salt method.

7   The ginger method uses a piece of ginger. Holes are **punched** in the ginger to allow the air and heat to **circulate**. Then the ginger is

较细的物质)

cone /kəʊn/ *n*.(实心或空心的)圆锥体

Lima bean /ˈliːmə biːn/ *n*.利马豆;青豆

punch /pʌntʃ/ *v*.拳打;以拳痛击

circulate /ˈsɜːkjəleɪt/ *v*.(液体

put on the patient's skin. The moxa is then put on the ginger and burned. If the pain becomes too severe for the patient, you can lift the moxa and ginger off the patient's skin until the patient is red and replace it. This method is mainly used in external medicine to relieve symptoms of cold, for instance, stomachache, diarrhea, and pain in the joints.

8   The second indirect method uses a **clove** of garlic. The garlic is cut into pieces, again making holes for the circulation of air, then put on the skin, just the same as the ginger. After four or five applications, change the garlic. The average number of application is five to seven per acupoint. This method is used for skin troubles, such as infections, tumors, and **carbuncles**. It is also used for **tuberculosis**

9   Another frequent method of moxibustion uses a combination of moxa, salt and ginger. The patient's **navel** is first filled with salt. Then ginger is placed on top. The moxa is then placed on the ginger and burned. This method is used for dysentery, acute **abdominal** pain, and symptoms of cold in the four limbs. The results of this method are often both fast and effective.

10   The **monkshood** method uses the Chinese monkshood which can either be placed on the skin like the ginger, or made into a small cake and then used. The procedure for the cake method is as follows: First cut the monkshood into pieces, then **pound** into powder. Combine with rice wine and form into a cake two to three mm thick. This cake is then placed on the skin, with the moxa placed on top of it. This method is especially good for the kidney because of the additional warmth it provides. It is also useful in surgery and for **ulcers** on the skin that will not heal.

11   Another special method combines acupuncture and moxibustion. Needles are **inserted** into the acupoints, then moxa is put on top of the needles. One of the benefits of this method is that heat can be **transmitted** by the needles, making the transmission of heat easier.

12   Another moxibustion method is called the cigar method. In this method the moxa is rolled up in paper, resembling a cigar. Then the cigar is **ignited** and moved up and down on or near the skin. This method is often used because it is convenient and effective. (928 words)

或气体)环流,循环

clove /kləʊv/ *n*. 蒜瓣

Carbuncle /ˈkɑːbʌŋkl/ *n*. 痈;疔
tuberculosis /tjuːˌbɜːkjuˈləʊsɪs/ *n*. 结核病
navel /ˈneɪvl/ *n*. 肚脐;脐

abdominal /æbˈdɒmɪnl/ *adj*. 腹部的
monkshood /ˈmʌŋkshʊd/ *n*. 附子植物

pound /paʊnd/ *v*. 反复击打; 连续砰砰地猛击

ulcer /ˈʌlsə(r)/ *n*. 溃疡

insert /ɪnˈsɜːt/ *v*. 插入;嵌入
transmit /trænzˈmɪt, trænsˈmɪt/ *v*. 传(热、声等);透(光等); 使通过

ignite /ɪgˈnaɪt/ *v*. (使)燃烧, 着火;点燃

Notes：

1. in season 应时的，当令
2. The size of the moxa cone and the number of applications that must be used will differ, depending on the severity of disease. 艾炷的大小和施灸的次数因疾病的严重程度而有所不同。
3. the rule of thumb 经验法则
4. the blister-producing method 瘢痕灸
5. the non-blister-producing method 无瘢痕灸

Task One　Reading Comprehension

1. Moxibustion is a therapy which uses _____ to blister the skin or to make the skin warm.

　　A. fire　　　　　　B. moxa　　　　　　C. leaves　　　　　　D. needle

2. The most common form of moxibustion is _____.

　　A. burning a piece of moxa on or near the skin

　　B. burning a piece of moxa on a cake

　　C. using a clove

　　D. using a garlic

3. The indirect method, unlike the direct method _____.

　　A. directly burn the moxa

　　B. does not burn the moxa

　　C. does not burn the moxa directly on the skin

　　D. does not indirectly burn the moxa

4. Which of the following is NOT true concerning the use of ginger method?

　　A. It can be used to stomach.

　　B. It can be used to treat diarrhea.

　　C. It can be used to relieve high fever.

　　D. It can be used to relieve pain in the joints.

5. In the sentence "Then the cigar is ignited and moved up and down on or near the skin" (line 2, last paragraph) the word "ignite" means _____.

　　A. cognize　　　　B. ignore　　　　　C. start to burn　　　　D. neglect

Task Two　Vocabulary

1. **Directions：Complete the following phrases respectively according to its corresponding meaning or equivalent in Chinese within the brackets.**

　1) _____（使……起泡）the skin

　2) _____（筛出）dirt

　3) _____（艾炷）method

　4) _____（金字塔形）piles of moxa

5) _____（相对）healthy

6) the_____（开始）stage of a disease

7) a _____（慢性的）illness

8) _____（多肉的）areas

9) the _____（瘢痕）method

10) the_____（无瘢痕）method

11) allow the air and heat to _____（循环）

12) _____（外的）medicine

13) _____（减轻）symptoms of cold

14) a_____（蒜瓣）of garlic

15) a _____（组合）of moxa, salt and ginger

16) the _____（严重性）of disease

17) _____（击打）into powder

18) heat can be _____（传送）

19) the _____（传导）of heat

20) _____（方便）and effective

2. Fill in the blanks with the words from the box and change the form when necessary.

comparative	application	severity	chronic	fleshy
punch	crumble	ignite	combination	abdominal
symptom	effective	procedure	transmit	convenient

1) But the medical community still needs a more _____, less expensive, less "invasive" way to diagnose Alzheimer's.

2) He looked much healthier than I remembered, his toasted almond（杏仁）face round and _____.

3) McGee's father said that hearing the diagnosis for his child was like getting _____ in the stomach.

4) Concerned with the climate change models that predicted that forest fires would increase in _____ and frequency, Flegal decided to research whether lead was going back into the atmosphere.

5) In 2016 the Centers for Disease Control and Prevention issued a guideline, reminding doctors that the drugs should be used only as a last resort for _____ pain.

6) Possible signs of accidental swallowing in children may include _____ pain, vomiting and fever.

7) Lockdown measures and travel restrictions were put into place _____ earlier than other nations.

8) All are concerned with different _____ of computer science to biomedicine.

9) As always, we encourage parents and guardians to keep their students home if they are

exhibiting flu-related _____.

10) Deforestation tends to divide large patches of forest into smaller fragments—where wildfires are more likely to _____ in the first place.

11) Changing one's habits and lifestyle may be a more _____ way to save money and, at the same time, prevent adverse drug effects.

12) But more than a thousand years after the Western Roman Empire _____ to dust, its concrete structures are still standing.

13) The authors fed the mice different _____ of fiber sources as part of their diet.

14) A 7-year-old British girl is credited with saving her mother's life with CPR (cardiopulmonary resuscitation, 心肺复苏) after learning how to perform the emergency _____ by watching videos on YouTube.

15) The parasite, also called a pork tapeworm (猪肉绦虫), is _____ to humans through consuming raw or undercooked beef or pork.

Task Three Writing

Please rewrite the text in a form of abstract (about 150 words)

Terminology

Basic TCM Terminology of Acupuncture and Moxibustion

Terminology	WHO	WFCMS
补泄	supplementation and draining	reinforcement and reduction
合谷刺	join valley needling	triple directional needling
恢刺	relaxing needling	lateral needling
扬刺	shallow surround needling	central-square needling
傍针刺	proximate needling	straight and side needling
刺络法	pricking bloodletting method	collateral pricking
电针仪	electro-acupuncture device	electric stimulator
温和灸	gentle moxibustion	mild moxibustion
雀啄灸	pecking sparrow moxibustion	sparrow-pecking moxibustion
灯火灸	juncibustion	burning-rash moxibustion
太乙神针	taiyi moxa stick moxibustion	taiyi miraculous moxa stick
雷火神针	thunder-fire wonder moxibustion	thunder-fire miraculous moxa stick
温针疗法	warm needling therapy	warming needle moxibustion
穴;腧穴;穴位	acupuncture point	acupuncture point; acupoint

continued

Terminology	WHO	WFCMS
经穴	meridian point	meridian/ channel point
五输穴	five transport points	five transport points
井穴	well point	well point
荥穴	brook point	brook point
输穴	stream point	stream point
经穴	river point	river point
合穴	sea point	sea point
郄穴	cleft point	cleft point
六腑下合穴	lower sea points of the six bowels	lower sea points of six *fu*-organs
背俞穴;俞穴	transport point	back transport point
八脉交会穴	confluence points of the eight vessels	confluence points of eight extraordinary meridians/channels
下合穴	lower sea points of the six bowels	lower sea point
络穴	connecting point	connecting point
原穴	source point	source point
特定穴	specific point	specific point
募穴	alarm point	alarm point
腹募穴	alarm point	alarm point of abdomen
八会穴	eight meeting points	eight meeting points
交会穴	crossing point	crossing point
阿是穴;天应穴	ouch point	ashi point
经外奇穴	extra point	extra point
奇穴	extra point	extra point
耳穴	ear point	ear point

本书配套数字教学资源

微信扫描二维码，加入中医英语
读者交流圈，获取配套教学视
频、学习课件、课后习题和沟通交
流平台等板块内容，夯实基础知识

The sages did not treat those already ill, but treated those not yet ill.

是故圣人不治已病,治未病①

Unit 10　Clinical Application of TCM

Warming-up

Before you listen（Watch）

In this section you will hear a short passage about "The Lung System and Lung *Qi* Deficiency Diagnosis". The following words and phrases may be of help.

correspond /ˌkɒrɪˈspɒndens/	*v.*	相符,相当
trustworthy /ˈtrʌs(t)wəːðɪ/	*adj.*	值得信任的
dependable /dɪˈpɛndəb(ə)l/	*adj.*	可靠的,可信赖的
tendency /ˈtɛnd(ə)nsɪ/	*n.*	倾向,趋势
recommendation /ˌrɛkəmɛnˈdeɪʃ(ə)n/	*n.*	推荐
broccoli /ˈbrɒkəlɪ/	*n.*	西兰花
mucus /ˈmjuːkəs/	*n.*	黏液

While you listen（Watch）

Listen to the passage carefully and fill in each of the blanks marked from 1) to 10) according to what you have heard.

　　The lung system in Chinese medicine includes the organ and the meridian. In the five elements, it corresponds to metal. In TCM personality, it is the person that is trustworthy and dependable. The lung functions in Chinese medicine include controlling the immune system and acting as a shield, a defense to stop external 1) _____ from invading the body. It regulates water 2) _____ to prevent retention. It opens into the nose for better breathing. It also manifests on the skin and body hair. Having clear, beautiful skin is a sign of a healthy lung system. It is in charge of respiration, as well as controlling the flow of *qi* in all the 3) _____ . And

---

① 《素问·四气调神大论篇》,Paul U. Unschuld 译。

finally, it controls the mind and body connection in order to keep the lung healthy. And in balance, we need to practice deep breathing exercise such as meditation, and avoiding smoking or constantly 4) _____ chemicals. But balance can be restored with acupuncture, herbal medicine, a good 5) _____ , Tai Chi, or Qigong.

Lung *qi* deficiency is a Chinese medicine pattern in diagnosis and is defined by the following symptoms. This patient has tendency to catch colds and flu often takes a long time to recover and has a poor 6) _____ system. Other symptoms may include environmental allergies, such as dust, animal vendors, pollen and hay fever. There may be a weak voice, 7) _____ and a pale tongue when it comes to treatment for lung *qi* 8) _____ . In Chinese medicine, licensed 9) _____ will use specific points for each patient and add LU 7 and ST 36 to tonify lung *qi*. And since food is medicine, here are the recommendations to 10) _____ lung *qi*. It is a good idea to incorporate more cooked broccoli and yams into the diet, as well as garlic and apples, and especially avoiding mucus-forming food such as dairy and sugar.

After you listen(Watch)

Please discuss with your partner the following questions and give your presentation to the class.

1) What is the function of lung in terms of physiology in TCM?

2) How can we keep balance of the lung system?

3) What are the symptoms of lung *qi* deficiency?

4) What is a good diet for lung *qi*?

Reading

 Text A

BEFORE CLASS

1. Quest for Definition

Directions: Explore online the definitions of the following terms from Text A and prepare a unique one-minute oral presentation for your class.

1) chronic bronchitis

2) emphysema

3) Mahuang (*Herba Ephedrae*)

4) secondary symptoms

5) retained fluid

2. Text-based Activities

Directions: Read carefully the part of Text A that corresponds to your task, and then prepare a unique one-minute oral presentation for your class.

PERFORMANCE IN CLASS

Your Task

1) What were the patient's manifestations in his initial visit?

2) In what way did the patient improve in his second visit?

3) What were the formulas he was prescribed?

4) Why was Xiao Qinglong Tang effective on the patient?

5) What are the major points that should be borne in mind when we use Xiao Qinglong Tang?

Cold Fluid Retention in the Lung: A Case Record

1　Chai, male, aged 53. Initial visit on December 3rd, 1994.

2　A. Initial visit①

3　The patient suffered from cough and **panting** for more than ten years, worsened in winter and improved in summer. He was diagnosed as having **chronic** bronchitis or chronic **bronchitis** complicated with **emphysema** and was treated in several hospitals by both TCM and Western medicine without significant effect. His present clinical manifestations include panting, **oppressed** feeling in the chest, **shrugged** shoulders when breathing, and thin white sputum which became worsened at night. In the morning, the patient expectorated **copious** sputum with the symptoms of chills in the back, black complexion, moist and **glossy** tongue coating, and wiry pulse with slipperiness in the cun region.

4　*Syndrome differentiation*　Cold fluid retained in the body and upwardly invading the lung②.

5　*Treatment principle*　Warm the lung and stomach to **dispel** cold fluid.

6　*Formula*　Modified Xiao Qinglong Tang (Minor Blue Dragon Decoction)③

7　*Medicinals*

Mahuang	(Herba Ephedrae)	9 g
Guizhi	(Ramulus Cinnamomi)	10 g
Ganjiang	(Rhizoma Zingiberis)	9 g
Wuweizi	(Fructus Schisandrae)	10 g
Xixin	(Herba Asari)	6 g

---

　　①　Initial visit 初次就诊,首诊;second visit 二诊。

　　②　Cold fluid retained in the body and upwardly invading the lung：寒饮内伏,上射于肺。

　　③　Modified Xiao Qinglong Tang (Minor Blue Dragon Decoction)：也可作 Xiao Qinglong Tang with modification,小青龙汤加减。

Fa Banxia	(Rhizoma Pinelliae Praeparatum)	14 g
Baishao	(Radix Paeoniae Alba)	9 g
Zhi Gancao	(Radix Glycyrrhizae Praeparata)	10 g

8   B. Second visit

9   After taking 7 doses of the above formula, cough and panting were markedly improved, and **sputum** was reduced. The patient could sleep at night and felt no oppression in the chest. Then Guiling Wuwei Gancao Tang (*Cinnamon Twig*, *Poria*, *Schisandra Chinensis* and *Licorice Decoction*) plus Xingren (*SemaiPruni Armeniacae*), Fa Banxia (*Pinelliae Praeparatum*) and Ganjiang (*Rhizoma Zingiberis*) were used to strengthen healthy *qi* and dispel pathogenic factors①.

10   C. Comments

11   Xiao Qinglong Tang is a formula that is quite effective for cough and panting due to cold fluid retention. Zhang Zhongjing applied this formula to treat **thoracic** fluid retention with cold attack in the exterior, fluid retention below the heart and other symptoms like cough, dyspnea, panting and inability to lie down②. The condition of this case was marked by cough, panting, clear thin sputum, chills in the back, moist and glossy tongue coating due to failure of the lung *qi* to ascend and descend because of internal **disturbance** of the lung by cold fluid retention. In this formula, Mahuang (*Herba Ephedrae*) and Guizhi (*Ramulus Cinnamomi*) can dispel exterior pathogenic factors and stop panting; Ganjiang (*Rhizoma Zingiberis*) and Xixin (*Radix et Rhizoma Asari*) can warm the lung and stomach, resolve retained fluid and assist Mahuang (*Herba Ephedrae*) and Guizhi (*Ramulus Cinnamomi*) to dispel cold; Banxia (*Rhizoma Pinelliae*) can expel turbid phlegm, strengthen the stomach and resolve retained fluid; Wuweizi (*Fructus Schisandrae Chinensis*) can nourish the kidney water to astringe lung *qi*; Shaoyao (*Radix Paeoniae Lactiflorae*) can nourish *yin* blood, protect liver *yin*, and function as the **modifier** to the three medicinals of Mahuang (*Herba Ephedrae*), Guizhi (*Ramulus Cinnamomi*) and Xixin (*Radix et Rhizoma Asari*) to eliminate the pathogenic factor without damaging the healthy *qi*; Zhi Gancao (*Radix Glycyrrhizae Praeparata*) can replenish *qi*, harmonizes the middle and regulate all of the medicinals. That is why this formula can dispel cold pathogenic factor, resolve retained fluid, and smooth lung *qi*.

12   It should be pointed out that this formula is **drastic** in inducing diaphoresis. So inappropriate application of it may injure both *yin* and *yang*, consequently worsening the disease③. Therefore, the following points should be borne in mind in clinical practice.

---

①   strengthen healthy *qi* and dispel pathogenic factors: 正邪兼顾。

②   Zhang Zhongjing applied this formula to treat thoracic fluid retention with cold attack in the exterior, fluid retention below the heart and other symptoms like cough, dyspnea, panting and inability to lie down: 张仲景用此方治疗"伤寒表不解,心下有水气""咳逆倚息不得卧"等支饮为患。句中 apply ...表示"应用于,用于",如 to apply the theory to the practice,把理论运用于实践。

③   It should be pointed out that this formula is drastic in inducing diaphoresis. So inappropriate application of it may injure both *yin* and *yang*, consequently worsening the disease: 应当指出的是,本方为辛烈发汗之峻剂,用之不当,每有伐阴动阳之弊,使病情加重。It should be pointed out that ... 应当指出的是。

13　Differentiation of complexion: Retained cold fluid is a *yin* pathogenic factor that usually damages *yang qi*, making the movement of both the nutritive and defensive *qi* sluggish and unable to reach the face①. That was why there appeared the symptoms of black complexion known as "water color (Shui Se)", or dark rings around the eyes known as "water ring (Shui Huan)", or dark patches on the forehead, bridge of nose, cheeks and chin, known as "water patch (Shui Ban)"②.

14　Differentiation of cough and panting: There are several conditions to be differentiated, such as severe cough with mild panting, severe panting with mild cough, simultaneous severe cough and panting, or failure to lie down, usually aggravated at night.

15　Differentiation of phlegm: As cold stagnates in the lung (metal) and *yang* deficiency results in fluid condensation, it will lead to production of phlegm and retained fluid. The sputum expectorated is often white and thin, or frothy and watery when spit on the ground, or looking like egg white with cool feeling.

16　Differentiation of tongue manifestation: As cold pathogenic factor injuries lung *qi* and the retained fluid congeals, the tongue coating is commonly moist and glossy with no obvious change of the tongue body. But if *yang qi* is impaired, the tongue will become pale, tender and enlarged.

17　Differentiation of pulse manifestation: As cold fluid retains in the body, the pulse usually appears wiry. If cold attacks exteriorly and fluid retains interiorly, the pulse will be floating and wiry, or floating and tight. If the disease is long standing with retention of cold fluid, the pulse is usually deep③.

18　Differentiation of secondary symptoms: Retained fluid in the body often moves with *qi* movement, leading to many secondary symptoms, such as dysphagia due to cold fluid obstructing *qi*, vomiting due to cold fluid attacking the stomach, dysuria due to cold fluid obstructing the lower, and edema due to cold fluid flowing into the four limbs. If the exogenous cold cannot be eliminated, *qi* of taiyang will stagnate, leading to fever and headache.

19　The above six points in identifying syndromes are objective indications for correct use of Xiao Qinglong Tang.

20　In this prescription, Fuling (*Sclerotium Poriae Cocos*), Xingren (*Semen Pruni Armeniacae*) and Shegan (*Rhizoma Belamcandae*) are added to strengthen the curative effect. Xiao Qinglong Tang is an efficacious formula for cough and panting due to cold fluid retention, but its action is so

---

①　making the movement of both the nutritive and defensive *qi* sluggish and unable to reach the face: 使荣卫行涩, 不能上华于面。

②　That was why there appeared the symptoms of black complexion known as "water color (Shui Se)", or dark rings around the eyes known as "water ring (Shui Huan)", or dark patches on the forehead, bridge of nose, cheeks, and chin, known as "water patch"(Shui Ban): 因而患者表现面色黧黑, 称为"水色"; 或两目周围有黑圈环绕, 称为"水环"; 或头额、鼻柱、两颊、下巴处出现黑斑, 称为"水斑"。

③　As cold fluid retains in the body, the pulse usually appears wiry. If cold attacks exteriorly and fluid retains interiorly, the pulse will be floating and wiry, or floating and tight. If the disease is long standing with retention of cold fluid, the pulse is usually deep: 寒饮之邪内停, 其脉多见弦象, 因弦主饮病; 如果是表寒里饮, 则脉多为浮弦或见浮紧; 若病久日深, 寒饮内伏, 其脉则多见沉。

strong in **dispersion** that it may consume lung *qi* in the upper, and affect kidney *qi* in the lower. If a patient with deficient healthy *qi* is improperly treated with this formula, side effects like severe cold limbs, feeling of *qi* rushing from the lower abdomen up to the chest and throat, and flushed face will be caused. This formula therefore must be discontinued as long as it effects a cure and cannot be taken for a long time. (1,063 words)

New Words and Expressions

pant /pænt/ *v.* to breathe rapidly in short gasps, as after exertion 气喘,喘

bronchitis /brɒŋ'kaɪtɪs/ *n.* chronic or acute inflammation of the mucous membrane of the bronchial tubes; a disease marked by this inflammation 支气管炎

emphysema /ˌemfɪ'siːmə/ *n.* a pathological condition of the lungs marked by an abnormal increase in the size of the air spaces; an abnormal distention of body tissues caused by retention of air 肺气肿;气肿

oppress /ə'pres/ *vt.* to keep down by severe and unjust use of force or authority; to weigh heavily on; to cause to suffer 压迫;压抑;抑制;使难受

shrug /ʃrʌg/ *v.* to raise (the shoulders), especially as a gesture of doubt, disdain, or indifference 耸肩

copious /'kəʊpɪəs/ *adj.* yielding or containing plenty; large in quantity; abundant 丰富的,多产的,大量的

glossy /'glɒsɪ/ *adj.* having a smooth, shiny, lustrous surface; superficially and often speciously attractive 平滑的,有光泽的

dispel /dɪs'pel/ *vt.* to rid one's mind of; to drive away or off by or as if by scattering 驱散,驱逐,使消散

sputum /'spjuːtəm/ *n.* a mixture of saliva and mucus coughed up from the respiratory tract, typically as a result of infection or other disease and often examined microscopically to aid medical diagnosis 痰

disturbance /dɪ'stɜːbəns/ *n.* the act of disturbing; the condition of being disturbed; something that disturbs, as a commotion, scuffle, or public tumult 骚动,动乱,打扰,干扰

thoracic /θɔː'ræsɪk/ *adj.* relating to the chest 胸的

modifier /'mɒdɪfaɪə(r)/ *n.* an agent that changes the form or characteristic of an object or substance 修饰成分

drastic /'dræstɪk/ *adj.* severe or radical in nature; extreme; taking effect violently or rapidly 激烈的,(药性等)猛烈的

patch /pætʃ/ *n.* a small piece, part, or section, especially that which differs from or contrasts with the whole 片,碎片,斑纹,斑点

simultaneous /ˌsɪm(ə)l'teɪnɪəs/ *adj.* occurring, operating, or done at the same time 同时发生

condensation /ˌkɒnden'seɪʃn/ *n.* water which collects as droplets on a cold surface when humid air is in contact with it 凝结

frothy /'frɒθɪ/ *adj.* full of or covered with a mass of small bubbles 有泡沫的

congeal /kənˈdʒiːl/ v. become semi-solid, especially on cooling 凝结

wiry /ˈwaɪərɪ/ adj. resembling wire in form and texture 像弦一样的

indicate /ˈɪndɪkeɪt/ vt. to show the way to or the direction of; point out; to serve as a sign, symptom; signify 指出,显示,象征

efficacious /ˌefɪˈkeɪʃəs/ adj. producing or capable of producing a desired effect 有效的,灵验的

dispersion /dɪˈspəːʃ(ə)n/ n. the action or process of distributing things or people over a wide area 分散

FOLLOW-UP ACTIVITIES

Task one   Comprehension Check

1. Questions for Discussion

1) How should we distinguish the symptoms of using Xiao Qinglong Tang from other formulas?

2) What are the pulse manifestations of retention of cold fluid?

3) What kind of patients should not be given Xiao Qinglong Tang?

4) How do you understand Zhang Zhongjing's application of Xiao Qinglong Tang?

2. Chart Completion

INITIAL VISIT: (para. 1 – 7)

The patient with cough and panting for more than ten years was diagnosed with 1) _____ _____ . Present examinations found 2) _____ _____ .

According to syndrome differentiation, he was of cold fluid retained in the body and upwardly invading the lung, so the treatment principle was to 3) _____ and 4) _____ was prescribed as the basic formula.

SECOND VISIT: (para. 8 – 9)

After taking 7 doses, the patient was markedly released from 5) _____ _____ and could sleep at night and felt no more oppression in the chest. The formula of 6) _____ and herbs like 7) _____ were used to strengthen healthy *qi* and dispel pathogenic factors.

COMMENTS: (para. 10 – 20)

In Xiao Qinglong Tang, Mahuang (*Herba Ephedrae*) and Guizhi (*Ramulus Cinnamomi*) are used to 8) _____ ; Ganjiang (*Rhizoma Zingiberis*) and Xixin (*Radix et Rhizoma Asari*) can 9) _____ ;Banxia (*Rhizoma Pinelliae*) can 10) _____ ; Wuweizi (*Fructus Schisandrae Chinensis*) can 11) _____ ; Shaoyao (*Radix Paeoniae Lactiflorae*) can 12) _____ and also modifies the other three medicinals; Zhi Gancao (*Radix Glycyrrhizae Praeparata*) can 13) _____ _____ .

There are 6 objective indications for correct use of Xiao Qinglong Tang.(1) to distinguish complexion, because 14) _____ ;

(2) to distinguish cough and panting, because 15) _____;
(3) to distinguish phlegm, because 16) _____;
(4) to distinguish tongue, because 17) _____;
(5) to distinguish pulse, because 18) _____;
(6) to distinguish secondary symptoms because 19) _____;

Xiao Qinglong Tang's action is strong in dispersion. If a patient with deficient healthy *qi* is improperly treated with this formula, there might be side effects such as 20) _____.

Task Two   Vocabulary

1. **Directions: Complete the following phrases respectively according to its corresponding meaning or equivalent in Chinese within the brackets.**

1) _____ feeling（憋闷）
2) _____ shoulders（耸肩）
3) _____ in the exterior（伤寒表不解）
4) _____ tongue coating（舌苔水滑）
5) exterior _____ factor（表邪）
6) stop _____ （平喘）
7) _____ cold（散寒）
8) _____ phlegm（痰浊）
9) _____ the stomach（健胃）
10) nourish the _____ （滋肾水）
11) _____ *qi*（荣气）
12) _____ lung *qi*（敛肺气）
13) _____ *qi*（卫气）
14) _____ complexion（面色黧黑）
15) _____ tongue（舌质淡嫩）
16) _____ tongue（舌体胖大）
17) _____ （轻微的）panting
18) severe _____ （手足厥冷）
19) _____ face（翕热如醉状）
20) _____ （舌苔）
21) _____ in the back（背部恶寒）
22) cold fluid _____ into the four limbs（饮溢四肢）
23) _____ differentiation（辨证论治）
24) _____ symptoms（次要症状）
25) treatment _____ （治则）
26) tongue _____ （舌体）
27) strengthen _____ *qi*（扶正）
28) water _____ （水斑）
29) water _____ （水色）
30) water _____ （水环）

2. **Match the following words with their proper meanings.**

Column I	Column II
1) disturbance	a. the act of disturbing; the condition of being disturbed; something that disturbs, as a commotion, scuffle, or public tumult
2) sputum	b. occurring, operating, or done at the same time
3) frothy	c. as a result
4) slipperiness	d. a mixture of saliva and mucus coughed up from the respiratory tract, typically as a result of infection or other disease and often examined microscopically to aid medical diagnosis
5) aggravate	e. to make worse or more troublesome

continued

Column I	Column II
6) consequently	f. difficulty or discomfort in swallowing, as a symptom of disease
7) inappropriate	g. slow-moving or inactive
8) sluggish	h. cease from doing or providing (something), especially something that has been provided on a regular basis
9) modifier	i. become semi-solid, especially on cooling
10) simultaneous	j. severe or radical in nature; extreme; taking effect violently or rapidly
11) congeal	k. able to cure disease
12) dysphagia	l. not suitable or proper in the circumstances
13) drastic	m. full of or covered with a mass of small bubbles
14) curative	n. the quality or state of being slippery
15) discontinue	o. an agent that changes the form or characteristic of an object or substance

3. Fill in the blanks with the words from the box and change the form when necessary.

simultaneous	oppress	curative	dysphagia	disturbance
bronchitis	discontinue	slipperiness	inappropriate	sputum
drastic	congeal	sluggish	efficacious	pant

1) She also cares about social justice, the plight (苦难) of the _____ and lots of other things.

2) The back of the throat and the lining (内层) of the windpipe may also slough off (蜕皮), and the dead tissue slides down the windpipe into the lungs or is coughed up with _____ .

3) In this he appeals to the medical profession for a trial of the _____ effects of electricity, and records many alleged cures.

4) It was a month of icy _____ , Arctic air and wintry precipitation (降水) that prompted the federal government to close early Tuesday and open late Wednesday.

5) "Parents and doctors should pay attention. These vaccines are highly _____ ," Wheeler said.

6) That email says that attorneys found that Gill used "_____ and unprofessional" language and that the campaign was taking steps to "remedy" the situation.

7) His breath hadn't caught up and he _____ from the climbing.

8) At home, the government faces a slowing economy, which is growing at its most _____ pace in 30 years, raising fears about unemployment.

9) The state took _____ measures that stirred a backlash, including creating a containment zone.

10) Experiences like these _____ fill me with hope and despair.

11) The elderly, young and people with weakened immune systems are at a higher risk of developing acute problems, such as _____ and pneumonia, according to the Centers for Disease Control and Prevention.

12) An estimated 9 million Americans suffer from difficulty swallowing, otherwise known as "_____".

13) Sleep _____ is also a feature of many psychiatric (精神病的) disorders, from depression to schizophrenia (精神分裂症).

14) The gruel was grey and watery, and he pushed it away after his third spoonful and let it _____ in the bowl.

15) You shouldn't _____ medications without checking with your doctor.

Task Three   Translation

1   Translate the following medical expressions into English

1) 首诊
2) 咳喘
3) 寒饮内伏
4) 正邪兼顾
5) 不得卧
6) 背部恶寒
7) 痰质清稀
8) 祛邪而不伤正
9) 调和诸药
10) 发汗
11) 水斑
12) 阳虚
13) 虚人
14) 少腹
15) 肺气
16) 面色黧黑
17) 有效方剂
18) 益气和中
19) 临床运用
20) 心下有水气

2   Translate the following sentences into Chinese or English

1) His present clinical manifestations include panting, oppressed feeling in the chest, shrugged shoulders when breathing, and thin white sputum which became worsened at night.

2) Xiao Qinglong Tang is a formula quite effective for cough and panting due to cold fluid retention.

3) The condition of this case was marked by cough, panting, clear thin sputum, chills in the back, moist and glossy tongue coating due to failure of the lung *qi* to ascend and descend because of internal disturbance of the lung by cold fluid retention.

4) If cold attacks exteriorly and fluid retains interiorly, the pulse will be floating and wiry, or floating and tight. If the disease is long standing with retention of cold fluid, the pulse is usually deep.

5) This formula therefore must be discontinued as soon as it effects a cure and cannot be taken for a long time.

6) 值得铭记的是这些中药是为疫情而备。(bear in mind)

7) 这位患者已发热、咳嗽、气短、呕吐 1 周。(suffer from)

8) 他曾被诊断为气血两虚证。(be diagnosed as)

9) 需要指出的是,临床辨证论治是关键。(It should be pointed out that ...)

10) 误用药性竣烈的方子,会导致肺肾之气耗伤。(lead to)

3 **Translate the following passage into English**

小青龙汤为解表剂,具有解表散寒、温肺化饮的功效。主治外寒里饮证。症见恶寒发热,头身疼痛,无汗,喘咳,痰涎清稀而量多,胸痞,或干呕,或痰饮喘咳,不得平卧,或身体疼重,头面四肢浮肿,舌苔白滑,脉浮。临床用于治疗慢性阻塞性肺气肿、支气管哮喘、急性支气管炎、肺炎、百日咳、过敏性鼻炎等。

↘ Text B

Chinese Herbs and Fertility

1   Chinese herbs have a long history of use in aiding fertility. Records indicating herbal treatment of **infertility** and **miscarriage** date back to 200 A.D., including mention of formulas that are still used for those purposes today, in the famous medical text *Shang Han Lun*. The first book devoted solely to gynecology and obstetrics, *The Complete Book of Effective Prescriptions for Diseases of Women*, was published in 1,237 A.D.

infertility /ˌɪnfɜːˈtɪlətɪ/ *n*. 不肥沃;贫瘠;不孕;不育
miscarriage /ˌmɪsˈkærɪdʒ/ *n*. 流产,小产

The herbs used to aid fertility

2   No individual herb is considered especially useful for promoting fertility. Rather, more than 150 different herbs, usually given in complex formulas comprised of 15 or more ingredients, are used in the treatment of infertility with the purpose of correcting a functional or organic problem that caused infertility. The design of the formulas has varied somewhat over the centuries, based on prevailing theories and available resources, and individual practitioners have a preference for particular herbs, thus accounting for some of the **variations** among formulas that are **recommended**. However, differences among individuals being treated accounts for the greatest variation in the selection of herbs and formulas to be used. There are some "exotic" materials that are frequently found in fertility formulas, such as deer **antler** and sea horse, but the prominent materials are derived from roots, **barks**, leaves, flowers, and fruits. Formulas for men and for women tend to be different, but there is considerable **overlap** in the ingredients used.

variation /ˌveərɪˈeɪʃn/ *n*.(数量、水平等的)变化,变更
recommend /ˌrekəˈmend/ *v*. 推荐;举荐;介绍
exotic /ɪɡˈzɒtɪk/ *adj*. 来自异国(尤指热带国家)的;奇异的;异国情调的;异国风味的
antler /ˈæntlə(r)/ *n*. 鹿角
bark /bɑːk/ *n*. 树皮
overlap /ˌəʊvəˈlæp/ *v*.(物体)部分重叠,交叠

The success rate for Chinese herb treatments

3   Although the outcome for any given individual cannot be

predicted, the clinical studies conducted in China indicate that about 70% of all cases of infertility (male and female) treated by Chinese herbs resulted in pregnancy or restored fertility. Depending on the particular study and the types of infertility treated, success rates ranged from about 50% up to more than 90%. Included in these statistics are cases of infertility involving obstruction of the **fallopian tubes**, amenorrhea, **absent ovulation**, **endometriosis**, **uterine fibroids**, low sperm count, nonliquification of **semen**, and other causes.

fallopian tube
/fəˌləʊpɪənˈtjuːb/ 输卵管
absent ovulation 排卵不足
endometriosis
/ˌɛndəʊˌmiːtrɪˈəʊsɪs/ n. 子宫内膜异位
uterine fibroids 子宫肌瘤
semen /ˈsiːmən/ n. 精液

Duration of treatment to attain fertility

4　In the Chinese clinical studies, daily or periodic use of herbs usually resulted in restored fertility within three to six months. Many Chinese doctors feel that if pregnancy is not achieved within about eight to nine months, then it is unlikely that the treatment will be successful with continued attempts. In Japan, where doctors give lower dosages of herbs and are restricted to using a smaller range of herbs, treatment time is usually longer: from six to fifteen months. In the U.S., nearly the full range of Chinese herb materials are accessible, but the dosage to be used is usually lower than in China; as a result, it is estimated that pregnancy can be achieved within six to twelve months. It must be remembered, however, that **approximately** one-third of infertility cases may fail to respond to all reasonable attempts. One advantage of the Chinese herbal **approach** is that even if pregnancy does not occur, benefits to health can be attained because the herbs address imbalances that affect other aspects of health besides infertility.

approximately
/əˈprɒksɪmətlɪ/ adv. 大概；大约；约莫
approach /əˈprəʊtʃ/ n. (待人接物或思考问题的)方式,方法,态度

Mechanism of action

5　The mechanism of action of the herbs is not known precisely, and undoubtedly varies according to the type of infertility problem being treated and the herb formula that is used. The traditional Chinese views are that infertility tends to arise from one or more of three **prominent** causes:

　　1) A "deficiency" syndrome prevents the **hormonal** system from properly influencing the sexual and **reproductive** functions. This is said to be a weakness of the "kidney and liver" which may influence various body functions producing symptoms such as frequent urination, weakness and aching of the back and legs,

prominent /ˈprɒmɪnənt/ adj. 重要的；著名的
hormonal /hɔːˈməʊnl/ adj. 荷尔蒙的
reproductive /ˌriːprəˈdʌktɪv/ adj. 生殖的；繁殖的

impotence, irregular **menstruation**, and difficulties with regulation of body temperature. Deficiency syndromes are treated with **tonic** herbs that are said to nourish *qi* (e.g. ginseng), blood (e.g. tang-kuei, ho-shou-wu), *yin* (e. g. **lycium fruit**), or *yang* (e. g. **epimedium**), and are selected according to the overall evaluation of symptoms.

　　2) A "**stagnancy**" syndrome prevents the sexual and reproductive organs from functioning despite normal hormone levels and normal ability to respond to hormones. This is said to involve a stagnancy of "*qi* and blood," which has the impact of restricting circulation to the tissues involved. *Qi* stagnation is often noted by tense muscles, restrained anger, and digestive disorders. Other symptoms that might arise include abdominal pain or bloating, **chronic** inflammation, and formation of lumps (including **cysts** and tumors). Blood stagnation often occurs following childbirth, surgery, injury, or severe infection and is typically noted when there is severe pain (such as dysmenorrhea), or hard swellings and obstructions; abnormal cell growth, including **dysplasia** and cancer, are thought to involve blood stagnation. Herbs such as **salvia**, **red peony**, and **carthamus** may be used.

　　3) A "heat" syndrome, which causes the affected organs to function abnormally. Heat syndromes may be associated with an infection or inflammatory process. This type of syndrome can produce abnormal semen quality leading to male infertility, while gynecologic infections can maintain female infertility by blocking the passages, altering the **mucous membrane** conditions, or influencing the local temperature. Herbs that inhibit infections and reduce inflammation are used, including **gardenia**, **phellodendron**, **patrinia**, and **lonicera**.

6　In each case, the purpose of the Chinese herbs is to **rectify** the underlying imbalance to restore normal functions. Western medicine can diagnose tubal blockage (which usually corresponds to blood stagnancy in Chinese medicine) and infection (which corresponds to heat syndromes of Chinese medicine) and in many cases can successfully treat these causes of infertility. However, Western medicine often fails to diagnose deficiency syndromes and most of the stagnancy syndromes. Therefore, the majority of Chinese herb formulas to be applied in the U.S. are those that **counteract** the deficiency (called tonics) and those that resolve the

---

impotence /'ɪmpətəns/ n. [泌尿][中医] 阳痿;虚弱

menstruation /ˌmenstru'eɪʃn/ n. 行经,月经来潮

tonic /'tɒnɪk/ n. 补药;滋补品

lycium fruit 枸杞子

epimedium /ˌepə'miːdjəm/ n. 淫羊藿,仙灵脾

stagnancy /'stægnənsɪ/ n. 停滞;迟钝;萧条;不景气

chronic /'krɒnɪk/ adj. 慢性的;难以治愈(或根除)的

cyst /sɪst/ n. 囊肿;囊;包囊

dysplasia /dɪs'pleɪzɪə/ n. 发育不良

salvia /'sælvɪə/ n. 鼠尾草

red peony n. 赤芍

carthamus n. 红花

mucous /'mjuːkəs/ adj. 黏液的;似黏液的;分泌黏液的

membrane /'membreɪn/ n. 膜

gardenia /gɑː'diːnɪə/ n. 栀子花

phellodendron /ˌfelə'dendrən/ n. 黄柏

patrinia n. 败酱草

lonicera /ləu'nɪsərə/ n. 忍冬;金银花

rectify /'rektɪfaɪ/ v. 矫正;纠正;改正

counteract /ˌkaʊntər'ækt/ v. 对……起反作用;抵消

stagnancy (called regulators).

Use of herbs when pregnancy occurs

7   The herbs for inducing fertility are usually discontinued once pregnancy is suspected or confirmed. In most cases, it is not necessary to use herbs during pregnancy. Women with a history of miscarriage or who are deemed at high risk for miscarriage (somewhat more common among women who have experienced prolonged infertility) may wish to take herbs that are traditionally used in such cases by Chinese women. Certain herbs can be used during pregnancy to enhance the health of the mother and to counteract symptoms of morning sickness. In addition, it is reported that labor can be made easier by proper application of herbs and acupuncture.

prolong /prə'lɒŋ/ *v*. 延长

Threatened miscarriage

8   Threatened miscarriage, if due to an imbalance in the mother's system (but not if due to genetic problems with the fetus), can often be overcome with application of herbs and possible adjunct therapy with moxa or acupuncture. The method to be used and the procedures to follow should be discussed early in the pregnancy so that appropriate steps can be taken should bleeding, fetal agitation, or early contractions occur. It is important to note that most cases of early miscarriage (sometimes called spontaneous abortion) are not related to an imbalance in the mother's system but are rather a natural and fairly common event, possibly due to a development problem of the embryo. Later in the pregnancy, weaknesses in the mother's system or excessive fetal movement, become a more prominent factor. There is a particular herb formula, called Tang-kuei and Peony Formula (*Dang Gui Shao Yao San*), which forms the basis of most treatments aimed at avoiding miscarriage but the formula is intended to be used mainly as a daily preventive therapy rather than an emergency treatment.

genetic /dʒə'netɪk/ *adj*. 遗传学的,基因的
fetus /'fiːtəs/ *n*. 胎儿

contraction /kən'trækʃn/ *n*. (肌肉的)收缩;(尤指分娩时的)子宫收缩

embryo /'embrɪəʊ/ *n*. 胚胎

Role of acupuncture

9   Chinese clinicians appear confident that most fertility problems can be overcome solely or primarily with the use of herbs; most medical books describing Chinese methods of treating infertility do not mention acupuncture. However, acupuncture therapy may

address particular symptoms of concern either directly related or unrelated to infertility, and might be influential in speeding up the development of normal fertility. In the event that infertility is mainly due to functional disorders, it is possible that acupuncture alone could resolve the problem. (1,327 words)

(adapted from http：// www.itmonline.org/arts/fertility.htm)

Notes：

1. Records indicating herbal treatment of infertility and miscarriage date back to 200 A.D., including mention of formulas that are still used for those purposes today, in the famous medical text *Shang Han Lun*. 本句主语为"records"，"indicating herbal treatment of infertility and miscarriage"为后置定语修饰"records"，谓语为"date back to"。另外，"that are still used for those purposes today"为定语从句修饰 formulas。

2. *The Complete Book of Effective Prescriptions for Diseases of Women*《妇人良方大全》

3. Mechanism of action：In pharmacology, the term mechanism of action（MOA）refers to the specific biochemical interaction through which a drug substance produces its pharmacological effect. "药物作用机制"，简称 MOA，指的是药物可以产生药理学效果的生化反应。

4. Therefore, the majority of Chinese herb formulas to be applied in the U.S. are those that counteract the deficiency (called tonics) and those that resolve the stagnancy (called regulators). 因此，大多数在美国使用的中医方药都用以治疗虚证(补益方药)以及用以祛瘀(调理方药)。

5. The herbs for inducing fertility are usually discontinued once pregnancy is suspected or confirmed. 一旦发现可能怀孕或怀孕成功，用以助孕的药通常会停用。

6. Threatened miscarriage 先兆性流产

7. The method to be used and the procedures to follow should be discussed early in the pregnancy so that appropriate steps can be taken should bleeding, fetal agitation, or early contractions occur. 在怀孕早期，医生都应就治疗方法及过程与当事人商讨，以便在孕期出血、胎儿躁动不安和孕早期宫缩等情况发生时采取适当的措施。从句中"should"表示"如果，万一"。

8. It is important to note that most cases of early miscarriage (sometimes called spontaneous abortion) are not related to an imbalance in the mother's system but are rather a natural and fairly common event, possibly due to a development problem of the embryo. 值得注意的是，大多数早期流产(有时称为自然流产)与母体身体系统失衡无关，而是一种自然的、相当普遍的现象，可能是由于胚胎的发育问题。

Task One　Reading Comprehension

1. According to the article, in which country the treatment time to attain fertility is the shortest?

    A. Japan　　　　　　B. the US　　　　　C. the UK　　　　D. China

2. According to the article, infertility can be caused by several reasons. Which one of the following is **NOT** mentioned in the article?

    A. "deficiency" syndrome　　　　　B. "cold" syndrome

    C. "stagnancy" syndrome   D. "heat" syndrome

3. What's the aim of the Chinese medicine in the treatment according to the article?

    A. to treat the illness that the patient contracts

    B. to rectify the underlying imbalance to restore normal functions

    C. to ease the nerves of the patient

    D. to alleviate pain of the patient

4. Which of the following is **NOT** correct?

    A. The first book devoted solely to gynecology and obstetrics is *The Complete Book of Effective Prescriptions for Females*.

    B. Most cases of early miscarriage are not related to an imbalance in the mother's system.

    C. Tang-kuei and Peony Formula (*Dang Gui Shao Yao San*) is intended to be used mainly as daily preventive therapy.

    D. Acupuncture might be influential in speeding up the development of normal fertility.

5. According to the article, in what circumstances herbs will be used during pregnancy?

    A. the pregnant mother suffered miscarriage or the pregnant mother is deemed at a high risk of miscarriage

    B. to enhance the health of the pregnant mother

    C. to counteract some certain symptoms

    D. All of the above

Task Two   Vocabulary

1. Directions: Complete the following phrases respectively according to its corresponding meaning or equivalent in Chinese within the brackets.

1) _____ infertility (助孕)   2) gynecology and _____ (产科)

3) _____ (盛行的) theories   4) chronic _____ (炎症,发炎)

5) _____ (生殖的) functions   6) _____ (阻塞) of the fallopian tubes

7) _____ (抵制) the deficiency   8) treatment of _____ (不孕)

9) _____ syndrome (瘀证)   10) female _____ (不孕)

11) functional _____ (紊乱)   12) _____ abortion (流产)

13) frequent _____ (尿频)   14) _____ herbs (补药)

15) _____ (囊肿) and tumors   16) _____ (内分泌的)system

17) to _____ (恢复) normal functions   18) the mucous _____ (膜)

19) to _____ (修正) the situation   20) absent _____ (排卵)

2. Fill in the blanks with the words from the box and change the form when necessary.

rectify	miscarriage	reproductive	exotic	estimate
agitation	obstetrics	impotent	prominent	recommend
genetic	infertility	prolong	ingredient	counteract

1）If we were to avoid having schedule overruns, we need to have only a small number of defects and quickly _____ any problems uncovered by tests.

2）The recovery is now two years old, yet job markets sputter, home prices continue plunging (骤降) and our leaders appear _____.

3）It reflects the fact that the new virus is a _____ relative of SARS-CoV, the virus responsible for the 2003 outbreak of severe acute respiratory syndrome.

4）We _____ that 42% of all breast cancers in the UK could be prevented through reducing alcohol consumption, exercise and weight control.

5）Several factors influence the _____ number, including how contagious the virus is, how susceptible people are, how many times people interact with each other, and how long those interactions last.

6）She brought her children into the world at a time when _____ was a primitive (原始的) art.

7）The three firms I am going to _____ are very competitive, and all very good.

8）This might mean building woodlots (林地) for local use, planting _____ species that grow faster and are worth more money alongside native ones, or creating nature reserves with associated tourism jobs.

9）Whenever a new virus emerges in the human species, scientists rush to quickly understand its unique structure and, hopefully, devise a vaccine to _____, or at least contain, it.

10）the situation is so stressful that pregnant women are experiencing early deliveries, _____ and low-birth weights.

11）Major depression and post-traumatic stress _____ are twice as prevalent (普遍的) in women, but tests designed to mimic (模仿) their symptoms in rodents (啮齿类动物) are typically developed and validated (验证) in males.

12）On 11 February, Zhong Nanshan, a _____ Chinese physician leading a panel of experts helping to control the outbreak, said that the coronavirus will possibly peak by the end of February.

13）Compounds from the plant and their derivatives (衍生物) are now _____ of numerous medications patented and sold by large pharmaceutical companies.

14）"We are still relatively ignorant about the causes of male _____, and as a matter of urgency we need to increase, substantially, our research effort into male reproductive health," said Barratt.

15）At the end of the 20th century the scientific research community has done wonders to fulfill medicine's historic goals of _____ life and alleviating suffering.

Task Three　Writing

Please rewrite the text in a form of abstract (about 150 words)

Terminology

Basic Terminology of TCM Clinical Application

Terminology	WHO	WFCMS
津	fluid	fluid/saliva
液	humor	thick liquid
肺气	lung *qi*	lung *qi*
肺气虚	lung *qi* deficiency	lung *qi* deficiency
症状	symptom	symptom
证	pattern/syndrome	pattern/syndrome
痰	phlegm	phlegm
饮;水饮	retained fluid	fluid retention; drink; decoction
痰饮	phlegm-retained fluid; phlegm-fluid retention	phlegm-fluid retention
饮证	fluid retention syndrome/pattern	fluid retention syndrome/pattern
舌体;舌质	tongue body	tongue texture
舌色	tongue color	tongue color
淡白舌	pale tongue	pale tongue
胖大舌	enlarged tongue	enlarged tongue
润苔	moist fur	moist coating
镜面舌	mirror tongue	mirror tongue
切脉	take the pulse	pulse taking and palpation
脉象	pulse condition	pulse manifestation
紧脉	tight pulse	tight pulse
辨证论治	pattern identification; syndrome differentiation and treatment	syndrome differentiation and treatment; pattern identification and treatment
治则	therapeutic principle	therapeutic principle
治法	method of treatment	therapeutic methods
解表散寒	release the exterior and dissipate cold	releasing exterior and dissipating cold
温肺化饮	warm the lung and resolve fluid retention	warming lung and resolving fluid retention
外寒	external cold	external cold; external cold manifestation
祛痰	dispel phlegm	dispelling phlegm
外邪;客邪	external pathogen	intruding pathogen
支饮	thoracic fluid retention	thoracic fluid retention

continued

Terminology	WHO	WFCMS
饮停胸胁证	pattern/syndrome of fluid retention in the chest and hypochondrium	syndrome/pattern of fluid retained in chest and hypochondrium
中草药	herbs; herbal drugs	Chinese herbal medicine
面黑	darkish complexion	blackish complexion
贮痰之器	receptacle that holds phlegm	container of phlegm
病位	location of disease	location of disease
病性	nature of disease	nature of disease
肺寒	lung cold	lung cold
肺虚	lung deficiency	lung deficiency
肾阴虚	kidney *yin* deficiency	kidney *yin* deficiency
肾阳虚；肾阳虚衰	kidney *yang* deficiency	kidney *yang* deficiency
肾气虚	kidney *qi* deficiency	kidney *qi* deficiency
体征	sign	sign
证型	pattern/syndrome type	syndrome/pattern type
司外揣内	judging the inside from observation of the outside	inspecting exterior to predict interior
四诊合参	correlation of all four examinations	comprehensive analysis of four examinations
八纲	eight principles	eight principles
主色	governing complexion	normal individual complexion
客色	visiting complexion	varied normal complexion
病色	morbid complexion	morbid complexion
善色	benign complexion	favorable complexion
恶色	malign complexion	unfavorable complexion
舌神	tongue spirit	tongue spirit
荣枯老嫩	luxuriant, withered, tough and tender-soft	flourishing, withered, tough and tender
脉象主病	disease correspondences of the pulse	diseases indicated by pulse conditions
热证	heat pattern/syndrome	heat syndrome/pattern
精气亏虚证	essential *qi* deficiency pattern/syndrome	essential *qi* deficiency syndrome/pattern
病因辨证	disease cause pattern identification/syndrome differentiation	disease cause syndrome differentiation/pattern identification
血瘀证	blood stasis pattern/syndrome	blood stasis syndrome/pattern
气滞血瘀证	pattern/syndrome of *qi* stagnation and blood stasis	syndrome/pattern of *qi* stagnation and blood stasis
寒痰阻肺证	pattern/syndrome of cold-phlegm obstructing the lung	syndrome/pattern of cold-phlegm obstructing lung

continued

Terminology	WHO	WFCMS
干咳	dry cough	dry cough
肺咳	lung cough	lung cough
月经不调	menstrual irregularities	menstrual irregularities
胎动不安	threatened abortion	threatened abortion
滑胎	habitual abortion	habitual abortion
堕胎	early abortion	early abortion; induced abortion
小产	late abortion	late abortion
过期不产	post-term pregnancy	post-term pregnancy
难产;产难	difficult delivery	difficult delivery
胎怯;胎弱	fetal weakness	fetal feebleness
宣肺	diffuse the lung	ventilating lung
宣肺化痰	diffuse the lung to resolve phlegm	ventilating lung and resolving phlegm
温肺化痰	warm the lung and resolve phlegm	warming lung and resolving phlegm
补法	tonifying method	tonifying method; tonification
安胎	prevent abortion	calming fetus; prevent abortion

本书配套数字教学资源

微信扫描二维码，加入中医英语
读者交流圈，获取配套教学视
频、学习课件、课后习题和沟通交
流平台等板块内容，夯实基础知识

Appendix Ⅰ　Excerpts from Translated Classics

1. 《素问·上古天真论篇》

原　　文	李照国译本	Unschuld 译本
昔在黄帝,生而神灵,弱而能言,幼而徇齐,长而敦敏,成而登天。	Huangdi, or Yellow Emperor, was born intelligent. He was eloquent from childhood. He behaved righteously when he was young. In his youth, he was honest, sincere and wise. When growing up, he became the Emperor.	In former times there was Huang Di. When he came to life, he had magic power like a spirit. While he was [still] weak, he could speak. While he was [still] young, he was quick of apprehension. After he had grown up, he was sincere and skillful. After he had matured, he ascended to heaven.
乃问于天师曰:余闻上古之人,春秋皆度百岁而动作不衰。	He asked Master Qibo, I am told that people in ancient times all could live for one hundred years without any signs of senility.	Now, he asked the Heavenly Teacher: I have heard that the people of high antiquity, in [the sequence of] spring and autumn, all exceeded one hundred years. But in their movements and activities there was no weakening.
今时之人,年半百而动作皆衰者,时世异耶? 人将失之耶?	But people nowadays begin to become old at the age of fifty. Is it due to the changes of environment or the violation of the way [to preserve health]?	As for the people of today, after one half of a hundred years, the movements and activities of all of them weaken. Is this because the times are different? Or is it that the people have lost this [ability]?
岐伯对曰:上古之人,其知道者,法于阴阳,和于术数,食饮有节,起居有常,不妄作劳,	Qibo answered, The sages in ancient times who knew the Dao (the tenets for cultivating health) followed [the rules of] Yin and Yang and adjusted Shushu (the ways to cultivate health). [They were] moderate in eating and drinking, regular in working and resting, avoiding any overstrain.	Qi Bo responded: The people of high antiquity, those who knew the Way, they modeled [their behavior] on yin and yang and they complied with the arts and the calculations. [Their] eating and drinking was moderate. [Their] rising and resting had regularity. They did not tax [themselves] with meaningless work.
故能形与神俱,而尽终其天年,度百岁乃去。	That is why [they could maintain a desirable] harmony between the Shen (mind or spirit) and the body, enjoying good health and a long life.	Hence, they were able to keep physical appearance and spirit together, and to exhaust the years [allotted by] heaven. Their life span exceeded one hundred years before they departed.

continued

原　文	李照国译本	Unschuld 译本
今时之人不然也,以酒为浆,以妄为常,醉以入房,以欲竭其精,以耗散其真,不知持满,不时御神,务快其心,逆于生乐,起居无节,故半百而衰也。	People nowadays, on the contrary, just behave oppositely. [They] drink wine as thin rice gruel, regard wrong as right, and seek sexual pleasure after drinking. [As a result,] their Jingqi (Essence-Qi) is exhausted and Zhenqi (Genuine-Qi) is wasted. [They] seldom [take measures to] keep an exuberance [of Jingqi] and do not know how to regulate the Shen (mind or spirit), often giving themselves to sensual pleasure. Being irregular in daily life, [they begin to] become old even at the age of fifty.	The fact that people of today are different is because they take wine as an [ordinary] beverage, and they adopt absurd [behavior] as regular [behavior]. They are drunk when they enter the [women's] chambers. Through their lust they exhaust their essence, through their wastefulness they dissipate their true [qi]. They do not know how to maintain fullness and they engage their spirit when it is not the right time. They make every effort to please their hearts, [but] they oppose the [true] happiness of life. Rising and resting miss their terms. Hence, it is [only] one half of a hundred [years] and they weaken.
夫上古圣人之教下也,皆谓之虚邪贼风,避之有时,恬惔虚无,真气从之,精神内守,病安从来。	When the sages in ancient times taught the people, they emphasized [the importance of] avoiding Xuxie (Deficiency-Evil) and Zeifeng (Thief-Wind) in good time and keep the mind free from avarice. [In this way] Zhenqi in the body will be in harmony, Jingshen (Essence-Spirit) will remain inside, and diseases will have no way to occur.	Now, when the sages of high antiquity taught those below, they always spoke to them [about the following]. The depletion evil and the robber wind, there are [specific] times when to avoid them. Quiet peacefulness, absolute emptiness the true qi follows [these states]. When essence and spirit are guarded internally, where could a disease come from?
是以志闲而少欲,心安而不惧,形劳而不倦,气从以顺,各从其欲,皆得所愿。故美其食,任其服,乐其俗,高下不相慕,其民故曰朴。	[Therefore people in ancient times all lived] in peace and contentment, without any fear. They worked, but never overstrained themselves, making it smooth for Qi to flow. [They all felt] satisfied with their life and enjoyed their tasty food, natural clothes and naive customs. [They] did not desire for high positions and lived simply and naturally.	Hence, the mind is relaxed and one has few desires. The heart is at peace and one is not in fear. The physical appearance is taxed, but is not tired. The qi follows [its appropriate course] and therefrom results compliance: everything follows one's wishes; in every respect one achieves what one longs for. Hence, they considered their food delicious, they accepted their clothes, and they enjoyed the common. Those of higher and those of lower status did not long for each other. The people, therefore, were called natural.
是以嗜欲不能劳其目,淫邪不能惑其心,愚智贤不肖不惧于物,故合于道。所以能年皆度百岁而动作不衰者,以其德全不危也。	That is why improper addiction and avarice could not distract their eyes and ears, obscenity and fallacy could not tempt their mind. Neither the ignorant nor the intelligent and neither the virtuous nor the unworthy feared anything. [Such a behavior quite] accorded with the Dao (the tenets for cultivating health). This is the reason why they all lived over one hundred years without any signs of senility. Having followed the tenets of preserving health, [they could enjoy a long life free from diseases].	Hence, cravings and desires could not tax their eyes. The excess evil could not confuse their hearts. The stupid and the knowledgeable, the exemplary and the non-exemplary, none was in fear of other beings. Hence, they were one with the Way. That by which all of them were able to exceed a lifespan of one hundred years, while their movements and activities did not weaken, [that was the fact that] their virtue was perfect and they did not meet with danger.

李照国.汉英对照 黄帝内经素问 [M].西安：世界图书出版西安公司,2005：3-5.

Unschuld, Paul U. *Huang Di nei jing su wen: an annotated translation of Huang Di's Inner Classic — Basic Questions*, University of California Press, Ltd. London, England, 2011：29-36.

2.《伤寒论》辨太阳病脉证并治上

原　　文	Mitchell, Ye, Wiseman 译本	罗希文译本
太阳之为病,脉浮,头项强痛而恶寒。	In disease of the greater yang, the pulse is floating, the head and nape are stiff and painful, and [there is] aversion to cold.	A floating pulse, headache, stiff neck, and a feeling of chill are always the general symptoms and sign of the Taiyang (Initial Yang) syndrome.
太阳病,发热,汗出,恶风,脉缓者,名为中风。	When in greater yang disease [there is] heat effusion, sweating, aversion to wind, and a pulse that is moderate, it is called wind strike.	The Initial Yang syndrome with symptoms and sign of fever, perspiration, chill and moderate pulse is termed febrile disease caused by Wind.
太阳病,或已发热,或未发热,必恶寒,体痛,呕逆,脉阴阳俱紧者,名为伤寒。	Greater yang disease, whether heat has effused or not, as long as there is aversion to cold, with generalized pain, retching counterflow, and yin and yang [pulses] both tight, is called cold damage.	The Initial Yang syndrome with or without fever, but with chill and pain in the body, nausea, vomiting and pulse tense both in Yin and Yang, is termed febrile disease caused by Cold (Shanghan).
伤寒一日,太阳受之,脉若静者,为不传;颇欲吐,若躁烦,脉数急者,为传也。	On the first day of cold damage, greater yang contracts [the disease]. If the pulse is tranquil, this means no passage; a strong desire to vomit, if [there is] agitation and vexation, and the pulse is rapid and urgent, means passage.	During the first day of febrile disease caused by Cold, the syndrome is at the Initial Yang Channel. If the pulse is quiet, the syndrome is not transmitting (into the next Channel). When the patient is restless and nauseated, and the pulse is speedy and mighty, then syndrome is transmitting.
伤寒二三日,阳明、少阳证不见者,为不传也。	When on the second or third day of cold damage, yang brightness and lesser yang signs are absent, it means no passage [has occurred].	During the first two or three days of febrile disease caused by Cold, if the symptoms of Greater Yang and Lesser Yang do not appear, then the syndrome is still at the Initial Yang Channel; it is not transmitting.
太阳病,发热而渴,不恶寒者,为温病。若发汗已,身灼热者,名曰风温。风温为病,脉阴阳俱浮,自汗出,身重,多眠睡,鼻息必鼾,语言难出。若被下者,小便不利,直视失溲;若被火者,微发黄色,剧则如惊痫,时瘛疭;若火熏之,一逆尚引日,再逆促命期。	When in greater yang disease [there is] heat effusion and thirst, without aversion to cold, [this] is warm disease. If, after sweating has been promoted, there is generalized scorching heat, this is called wind-warmth. [When] wind-warmth causes disease, the yin and yang pulses are both floating, [there is] spontaneous sweating, generalized heaviness, a tendency to sleep, the breath [from the] nose will [make a] snoring [sound], and speech is difficult. If precipitation has been used, [there is] inhibited urination, forward staring eyes, and fecal incontinence; if fire has been used, [there is] slight yellowing, and in acute cases [there is] fright epilepsy, periodic tugging and slackening, and [the skin] appears as if fumed by fire; one [instance of] of adverse [treatment] will lengthen the time [of disease], and further adverse [treatment] will lead to the term of life.	The Initial Yang syndrome with fever and thirst but without chill is termed acute febrile disease (Wenbing). After adoption of diaphoresis, if the patient feels a scorching heat in the body, it is termed acute febrile disease caused by Wind (Fengwen), which bears the symptoms and signs of floating pulse at Yin and Yang, perspiration, a heavy feeling in the movement of the limbs, a tendency to fall asleep and snore soundly, and difficulty in pronunciation. A dose of purgative will cause dysuria or incontinence of urine and a staring vision. If the patient is scorched for the purpose of diaphoresis, his skin first turns yellowish, and then convulsions and spasms will occur. After one incorrect treatment, there are still a few days left for a rescue. If the patient is scorched again, no time will be left for rescue.

continued

原　文	Mitchell, Ye, Wiseman 译本	罗希文译本
病有发热恶寒者,发于阳也;无热恶寒者,发于阴也。发于阳,七日愈;发于阴,六日愈。以阳数七,阴数六故也。	When an illness [is characterized by] heat effusion and aversion to cold, it is springing from yang; when [an illness is characterized by] the absence of heat effusion and [the presence of] aversion to cold, it is springing from yin. [In illness] springing from yang, [the patient] recovers in seven days. [In illness] springing from yin, [the patient] recovers in six days. This is because yang numbers seven and yin numbers six.	The syndrome with fever and chill comes from Yang and takes seven days to heal; that with chill but no fever comes from Yin and takes six days to heal. Seven is a Yang (odd) number and six is a Yin (even) number.
太阳病,头痛至七日以上自愈者,以行其经尽故也。若欲作再经者,针足阳明,使经不传则愈。	When in greater yang disease, a headache lasts for more than seven days, [and then the patient] spontaneously recovers, this is because [the evil] has gone right through the channel. If it is about to pass to another channel, and [one] needles the foot yang brightness to prevent passage, then [the patient will] recover.	Initial Yang syndrome: If headache subsides in more than seven days, it is because the syndrome has circulated through the Initial Yang Channel. If the syndrome tends to transmit into the next Channel (Greater Yang), then acupuncture on acupoints of the Stomach Channel of Foot Yangming (Greater Yang) will stop the transmission of Channels. Thus, the syndrome is gone.
太阳病欲解时,从巳至未上。	The time when greater yang disease is about to resolve is from si (B6) to wei (B8).	The Initial Yang syndrome subsides approximately between si and wei (Shichen).
风家,表解而不了了者,十二日愈。	Wind patients in whom the exterior has resolved, but not clearly, will recover in twelve days.	After the dispersion of the Exterior syndrome of a patient who is apt to catch febrile disease by Wind, it still takes twelve days for him to get rid of general malaise.
病人身大热,反欲得衣者,热在皮肤,寒在骨髓也;身大寒,反不欲近衣者,寒在皮肤,热在骨髓也。	When the patient has great generalized heat, but desires to put [more] clothes on, the heat is in the skin and the cold is in the bone marrow; when [there is] great generalized cold, but [the patient] has no desire for clothes, the cold is in the skin and the heat is in the bone marrow.	If the patient has a high fever but wishes to have more clothes on, it indicates "Cold in the marrow, but Heat on the skin"; if the patient feels a chill but wishes to remove clothing, it is "Heat in the marrow, but Cold on the skin."
太阳中风,阳浮而阴弱。阳浮者,热自发,阴弱者,汗自出。啬啬恶寒,淅淅恶风,翕翕发热,鼻鸣干呕者,桂枝汤主之。	In greater yang wind strike with floating yang and weak yin, floating yang is spontaneous heat effusion, and weak yin is spontaneous issue of sweat. If [there is] huddled aversion to cold, wetted aversion to wind, feather-warm heat effusion, noisy nose, and dry retching, Cinnamon Twig Decoction (gui zhi tang) governs.	The pulse of Initial Yang febrile disease caused by Wind is floating when felt at the surface and weak in depth. Floating at the surface signifies Heat; weak in depth signifies spontaneous perspiration. Prescribe Decoction of Ramulus Cinnamomi when the patient feels chill and fears wind, uneasy because of a fever, nauseous and with a tendency to snore.

Mitchell, C., Ye F., Wiseman, N. *Shang Han Lun On Cold Damage*, Paradigm Publications, Brooklyn, USA, 1999: 41 - 61, 135.
罗希文. 伤寒论[M].北京: 新世界出版社,2005: 1 - 5.

3.《金匮要略》五脏风寒积聚病脉证并治

原　文	Wiseman, Wilms 译本	李照国译本
问曰：三焦竭部，上焦竭善噫，何谓也？	Question："[Regarding] exhaustion of the triple burner in [its different] sections, exhaustion in the upper burner causes a tendency to belching. Why is that?"	Question：[There are cases where] the triple energizer has declined, [But when] the upper energizer [begins] to decline, [the patient] tends to sigh. What is the reason?
师曰：上焦受中焦气未和，不能消谷，故能噫耳。	The Master says："The upper burner receives [qi from] the center burner. If qi is not in harmony, it cannot disperse grain, hence there is belching.	The master said：[When] qi transmits from the upper energizer to the middle energizer and fails to harmonize, [the patient is] unable to digest food, and that is why there is frequent sighing.
下焦竭，即遗溺失便，其气不和，不能自禁制，不须治，久则愈。	Exhaustion in the lower burner causes enuresis and fecal incontinence. [The reason for this is that] if qi is not in harmony, it cannot by itself ensure continence. You do not need to treat this condition; [the patient] will recover over time."	[When] the lower energizer [begins] to decline, [it will] cause enuresis and incontinence of defecation. [Since] qi is not harmonized, [the patient is] unable to control [the movement] spontaneously. [There is] no need to treat it. [After] a certain period of enduring, [the disease will] heal spontaneously.
师曰：热在上焦者，因咳为肺痿；热在中焦者，则为坚；热在下焦者，则尿血，亦令淋秘不通。	The Master says："Heat in the upper burner results in coughing and because of this, lung wilting. Heat in the center burner results in hardness. Heat in the lower burner results in bloody urine and also causes strangury and stoppage.	Question：[When pathogenic] heat is in the upper energizer, [it will] cause cough and lung wilting; [when pathogenic] heat is in the middle energizer, it is hard; [when pathogenic] heat is in the lower energizer, [there will be] blood in urine and stranguria will be caused.
大肠有寒者，多鹜溏；有热者，便肠垢。小肠有寒者，其人下重便血；有热者，必痔。	Cold in the large intestine causes profuse duck's slop; heat there causes intestinal grime in the stool. Cold in the small intestine causes heaviness in the lower [body] and bloody stool; heat there invariably causes hemorrhoids."	[When] there is cold in the large intestine, [there will be] incessant sloppy stool; [when pathogenic] heat is in the large intestine, [there will be] sticky stool; [when pathogenic] cold is in the small intestine, the patient [will suffer from] tenesmus and bloody stool; [when] there is [pathogenic] heat [in the small intestine], hemorrhoids will be caused.
问曰：病有积、有聚、有䅽气，何谓也？	Question："What do the diseases accumulations, gatherings, and grain qi refer to?"	Question：[In] diseases, [there are] accumulations, gatherings and cereal qi. What are they?
师曰：积者，脏病也，终不移；聚者，腑病也，发作有时，展转痛移，为可治；䅽气者，胁下痛，按之则愈，复发为䅽气。	The Master says："Accumulations are a disease of the viscera; they never move. Gatherings are a disease of the bowels; they erupt intermittently, spread from place to place, and manifest with mobile pain; they can be treated. Grain qi is pain under the rib-side that is relieved by pressure; when it is recurrent, it is grain qi.	The master said：Accumulations [indicate] a disease of zang-organs that never moves; gatherings [indicate] a disease of fu-organs that occurs in a certain time and pain that moves and is curable; cereal qi [indicates] pain below the rib-side that is relieved when pressed, but returns [when it] becomes cereal qi.
诸积大法：脉来细而附骨者，乃积也。	The general method for diagnosing the various accumulations: A pulse that is fine on arrival and is fixed to the bone indicates accumulations.	The major method [used to diagnose] various accumulations：The pulse [that is] thin and fixed to the bone [when pressed] indicates accumulations.

continued

原　文	Wiseman, Wilms 译本	李照国译本
寸口,积在胸中;微出寸口,积在喉中;	When [this type of pulse occurs] at the inch opening, the accumulation is in the chest; when it is slightly outside the inch opening, the accumulation is in the throat;	[When the pulse in] cunkou [region is thin], the accumulation is in the chest; [when] the faint [pulse] moves outside cunkou, [it indicates that] the accumulation is in the throat;
关上,积在脐旁;上关上,积在心下;微下关,积在少腹;	when it is on the bar, the accumulation is beside the umbilicus; when it is above the bar, the accumulation is below the heart; when it is slightly below the bar, the accumulation is in the lesser abdomen;	[when the pulse is thin and moves to] the upper of guan [region], [it indicates that] the accumulation is in the heart; [when the pulse is] faint [and moves to] the lower of guan [region], [it indicates that] the accumulation is in the lower abdomen.
尺中,积在气冲;脉出左,积在左;脉出右,积在右;脉两出,积在中央,各以其部处之。	when it is in the cubit, the accumulation is in the qi thoroughfare. When [this type of] pulse appears on the left, the accumulation is on the left; when [this type of] pulse appears on the right, the accumulation is on the right; when it appears on both sides, the accumulation is in the middle. You can locate each according to the position [of this pulse]."	[When] chi [pulse is thin], the accumulation is in Qichong (ST 30). [When] the [thin] pulse moves to the left, the accumulation is in the left; [when] the [thin] pulse is in the right, the accumulation is in the right; [when] the [thin] pulse moves to both sides, the accumulation is in the center. [It] can be treated according to its location in different places.

Wiseman, N.; Wilms S. *Jin Gui Yao Lue Essential Prescriptions of the Golden Cabinet*, Paradigm Publications, Taos, New Mexico USA. 2013: 256 – 259.
李照国. 汉英对照 金匮要略 [M].上海:上海三联书店,2017: 246 – 250.

4.《难经》四十九难

原　文	Unschuld 译本
曰: 有正经自病,有五邪所伤,何以别之?	It happens that the regular conduits fall ill by themselves, or that one is harmed by any of the five evils. How can these [situations] be distinguished?
然: 经言忧愁思虑则伤心;形寒饮冷则伤肺;恚怒气逆,上而不下则伤肝;饮食劳倦则伤脾;久坐湿地,强力入水则伤肾。是正经之自病也。	It is like this. The scripture states: Grief and anxiety, thoughts and considerations harm the heart; a cold body and chilled drinks harm the lung; hate and anger let the influences flow contrary to their proper direction; they move upward but not downward. This harms the liver. Drinking and eating [without restraint], as well as weariness and exhaustion, harm the spleen. If one sits at a humid place for an extended period, or if one exerts one's strength and goes into water, that harms the kidneys. These are [examples of situations where] the regular conduits fall ill by themselves.
何谓五邪?	What is meant by "the five evils"?
然: 有中风,有伤暑,有饮食劳倦,有伤寒,有中湿。此之谓五邪。	It is like this. To be hit by wind, to be harmed by heat, to drink and eat [without restraint], as well as weariness and exhaustion, to be harmed by cold, to be hit by humidity, these [conditions] are called the five evils.
假令心病,何以知中风得之?	Let us take an illness in the heart as an example. How does one know that [the patient] has contracted it because he was hit by wind?
然: 其色当赤。何以言之? 肝主色,自入为青,入心为赤,入脾为黄,入肺为白,入肾为黑。肝为心邪,故知当赤色也。其病身热,胁下满痛,其脉浮大而弦。	It is like this. His complexion should be red. Why do I say so? The liver rules the colors. [The color it keeps] itself is virid. [The color that is generated when its influences] enter the heart is red. [The color that is generated when its influences] enter the spleen is yellow. [The color that is generated when its influences] enter the lung is white. [The color that is generated when its influences] enter the kidneys is black. Hence one knows from the red complexion [of a patient] that the liver has [sent its influences into] the heart, causing the presence of evil [influences there]. [The patient] will suffer from a hot body, and [he will perceive] fullness and pain below the ribs. [The movement of the influences in] his vessels is at the surface, strong, and stringy.

continued

原　　文	Unschuld 译本
何以知伤暑得之?	How does one know that [the patient has] contracted [his illness in the heart] because he was harmed by heat?
然:当恶焦臭。何以言之? 心主臭,自入为焦臭,入脾为香臭,入肝为臊臭,入肾为腐臭,入肺为腥臭。故知心病伤暑得之,当恶焦臭。其病身热而烦,心痛,其脉浮大而散。	It is like this. He should have a bad odor. Why do I say so? The heart rules the odors. [The odor that is generated by] itself is burnt. [The odor that is generated when the heart sends its influences] into the spleen is aromatic. [The odor that is generated when the heart sends its influences] into the liver is fetid. [The odor that is generated when it sends its influences] into the kidneys is foul. [The odor that is generated when it sends its influences] into the lung is frowzy. Hence one knows if an illness in the heart has been contracted because of harm caused by heat, there should be a bad odor. The patient will suffer from a hot body and will feel uneasy. He has heartaches, and [the movement in] his vessels is at the surface, strong, and dispersed.
何以知饮食劳倦得之?	How does one know that [the patient has] contracted [his illness in the heart] because of [unrestrained] drinking and eating, or because of weariness and exhaustion?
然:当喜苦味也。何以言之? 脾主味,入肝为酸,入心为苦,入肺为辛,入肾为咸,自入为甘。故知脾邪入心,为喜苦味也。其病身热而体重,嗜卧,四肢不收,其脉浮大而缓。	It is like this. He should prefer [to consume food with a] bitter taste. [When one's spleen is] depleted, one will not wish to eat; [when one's spleen] is replete, one will wish to eat. Why do I say so? The spleen rules [one's preferences for a specific] taste. [The taste one prefers when the spleen sends its influences] into the liver is sour. [The taste one prefers when the spleen sends its influences] into the heart is bitter. [The taste one prefers when the spleen sends its influences] into the lung is acrid. [The taste one prefers when the spleen sends its influences] into the kidneys is salty. [The taste one prefers when the spleen keeps its influences] within itself is sweet. Hence one knows that if evil [influences] from the spleen enter the heart, that causes a preference for bitter taste. The patient will suffer from a hot body; [he will perceive] his body to be heavy and will have a desire to lie down. He cannot contract his four limbs. [The movement in] his vessels is at the surface, strong and relaxed.
何以知伤寒得之?	How does one know that [the patient has] contracted [his illness in the heart] because of harm caused by cold?
然:当谵言妄语。何以言之? 肺主声,入肝为呼,入心为言,入脾为歌,入肾为呻,自入为哭。故知肺邪入心,为谵言妄语也。其病身热,洒洒恶寒,甚则喘咳,其脉浮大而涩。	It is like this. He should talk incoherently and utter nonsense. Why do I say so? The lung rules the sounds. [The influences it sends] into the liver [cause one] to call. [The influences it sends] into the heart [cause one] to speak. [The influences it sends] into the spleen [cause one] to sing. [The influences it sends] into the kidneys [cause one] to groan. [The influences it keeps] within itself [cause one] to wail. Hence one knows that if evil [influences] from the lung have entered the heart, they cause [the patient] to talk incoherently and to utter nonsense. The patient will suffer from a hot body, he will shiver, and he will dislike cold. In extreme cases, that leads to coughing. [The movement in] his vessels is at the surface, strong, and rough.
何以知中湿得之?	How does one know that [the patient has] contracted [his illness in the heart] because he was hit by humidity?
然:当喜汗出不可止。何以言之? 肾主液,入肝为泣,入心为汗,入脾为涎,入肺为涕,自入为唾。故知肾邪入心,为汗出不可止也。其病身热,而小腹痛,足胫寒而逆,其脉沉濡而大。此五邪之法也。	It is like this. He should have a tendency to sweat without end. Why do I say so? The kidneys rule the liquids. [The liquid that is generated when they send their influences] into the liver is tears. [The liquid that is generated when they send their influences] into the heart is sweat. [The liquid that is generated when they send their influences] into the spleen is saliva. [The liquid that is generated when they send their influences] into the lung is snivel. [The liquid that is generated when they keep their influences] within themselves is spittle. Hence one knows that if evil [influences] from the kidneys have entered the heart, that causes [the patient] to sweat without end. He will suffer from a hot body and from pain in the lower abdomen; his feet and shinbones will be cold, and [the influences will] move contrary to their proper course. [The movement in] his vessels is deep, soft, and strong. These are the patterns of the five evils.

Unschuld, Paul U. *Nan-Ching The Classics of Difficult Issues*, University of California Press, Ltd. London, England, 1986: 457 - 460.

5.《神农本草经》

原　文	李照国译文
甘草 味甘,平。 主五脏六腑寒热邪气,坚筋骨,长肌肉,倍力,金疮,尰,解毒。久服轻身延年(《御览》引云一名美草,一名密甘,《大观本》,作黑字)。生川谷。	[Gancao(甘草, licorice, Radix Glycyrrhea Praeparata),] sweet in taste [and] mild [in property], [is mainly used] to treat [disease caused by] pathogenic cold and heat in the five Zang-organs and six fu-organs, to strengthen sinews and bones, to promote muscles, to increase strength, to cure traumatic injury and swollen foot, and to resolve toxin. Long-term taking [of it will] relax the body and prolong life. [It grows in mountain valleys and river valleys.
柴胡 味苦平。 主心腹,去肠胃中结气,饮食积聚,寒热邪气,推陈致新。久服,轻身明目益精。一名地熏。	[Chaihu (柴胡, bupleurum, Radix Bulpeuri),] bitter in taste and mild [in property], [is mainly used] to treat [disorders of] the heart and abdomen, to eliminate binding of Qi in the intestines and stomach [as well as] accumulation of [undigested] food [in the stomach], to remove evil-Qi in cold and heat, and to get rid of the stale to bring forth the fresh. Long-term taking [of it will] relax the body, improve vision and replenish essence. [It is also] called Dixun (地熏).
细辛 味辛,温。 主咳逆,头痛,脑动,百节拘挛,风湿,痹痛,死肌。久服明目,利九窍,轻身长年。一名小辛,生山谷。	[Xixin (细辛, as arum, Herba Asari),] pungent in taste and warm [in property], [is mainly used] to treat cough with dyspnea, headache, head shaking, spasm of joints, wind-dampness impediment and pain, and numbness of muscles. Long-term taking [of it can] improve vison, disinhibit nine orifices, relax the body and prolong life. [It is also] called Xiaoxin (小辛), growing in mountains and valleys.
石斛 味甘,平。 主伤中,除痹,下气,补五脏虚劳,羸瘦,强阴。久服厚肠胃,轻身延年。一名林兰(《御览》引云,一名禁生,观本,作黑字),生山谷。	[Shihu (石斛, dendrobe, Herba Dendrobii), sweet in taste and mild [in property], [is mainly used] to treat internal damage, to eliminate impediment, [promote] Qi to descend, to tonify the five Zang-organs [to treat] deficiency [due to] overstrain and emaciation, and to strengthen Yin. Long-term taking [of it will] invigorate the intestines and stomach, relax the body and prolong life. [It is also] called (林兰), growing in mountains and valleys.
雄黄 味苦,平寒。 主寒热,鼠瘘恶创,疽痔死肌,杀精物,恶鬼,邪气,百虫毒,胜五兵。炼食之,轻食神仙。一名黄食石。生山谷。	[Xionghuang (雄黄, realgar；Realgar),] bitter in taste, mild and cold [in property], [is mainly used] to treat cold-heat [disease], atrophy [caused by scrofula], severe sore, carbuncle, hemorrhoids and putrescence of muscles, to expel [severe pathogenic factors like] monster and ghost, [and to eliminate] evil-Qi and all worm toxin. [It is] much better than five [kinds of important] weapons. To take refined Xionghuang (雄黄, realgar; Realgar) will enable people to relax the body [as dexterous as] immortals. [It is also] called Huangshishi (黄食石) and can be found in mountains and valleys.
石膏 味辛,微寒。 主中风寒热,心下逆气惊喘,口干,苦焦,不能息,腹中坚痛,除邪鬼,产乳,金创。生山谷。	[Shigao (石膏,gypsum, Gypsum Fibrosum),] pungent in taste and slightly cold [in property], [is mainly used] to treat [disease caused by pathogenic] wind, cold and heat, fright and panting [due to] upward counterflow of Qi from below the heart, dryness of the mouth with scorched tongue [as well as] stiffness and pain of the abdomen, to eliminate [pathogenic factors like] evil and ghost, to promote lactation and to cure injury [caused by] metal. [It] exists in mountains and valleys.
干姜 味辛,温。 主胸满咳逆上气,温中止血,出汗,逐风,湿痹,肠澼,下利。生者尤良,久服去臭气,通神明。生川谷。	[Ganjiang (干姜, dry ginger, Rhizoma Zingiberis),] pungent in taste and warm [in property], [is mainly used] to relieve chest fullness, cough with dyspnea and upward counterflow of Qi, to warm the middle (the internal organs), to cease bleeding, to promote sweating, to expel wind, to treat dampness impediment, dysentery and diarrhea. The raw one is more effective. Long-term taking [of it will] remove foul smell and invigorate spirit and mentality. [It] grows in mountain valleys and river valleys.

continued

原 文	李照国译文
麻黄 味苦,温。 主中风伤寒头痛温疟,发表,出汗,去邪热气,止咳逆上气,除寒热,破癥坚积聚。一名龙沙。	[Mahuang (麻黄, ephedra, Herba Ephedrae),] bitter in taste and warm [in property], [is mainly used] to treat wind stroke, headache, cold damage and malaria, to relieve superficies, to induce sweating, to eliminate evil-heat Qi, to stop cough with dyspnea with upward lump and accumulation [of pathogenic factors]. [It is also] called Longsha (龙沙).
芍药 味苦,平。 主邪气腹痛,除血痹,破坚积寒热,疝瘕,止痛,利小便,益气(艺文类聚引云:一名白术,《大观本》,作黑字)。生川谷及丘陵。	[Shaoyao (芍药, peony, Radix Paeoniae),] bitter in taste and mild [in property], [is mainly used] to expel evil-Qi, to relieve abdominal pain, to eliminate blood impediment, to dispel hard accumulation of cold and heat, to cease pain, to promote urination and to replenish Qi. [It] grows in mountain valleys, river valleys and hills.
附子 味辛,温。 主风寒咳逆邪气,温中,金创,破癥坚积聚,血瘕,寒温,踒(《御览》作痿)。躄拘挛,脚痛,不能行步(《御览》引云:为百药之长,《大观本》,作黑字)。生山谷。	[Fuzi (附子, aconite, Radix Aconiti Praeparata),] pungent in taste and warm [in property], [is mainly used] to relieve wind-cold [syndrome/pattern] and cough with dyspnea [caused by] evil-Qi, to warm the middle, [to heal] sore [caused by] metal, to eliminate obstinate conglomeration, accumulation and scabies, [to treat] abdominal mass with blood, limp and spasm of legs [due to] pain of the feet. [It] grows in mountains and valleys.

李照国.汉英对照 神农本草经 [M].上海:上海三联书店,2017: 86 - 87, 118 - 119, 154 - 155, 158 - 159, 526 - 527, 540 - 541, 570 - 571, 590 - 591, 598 - 599, 932 - 933.

6.《本草纲目》人参

原 文	罗希文译本
【主治】补五脏,安精神,定魂魄,止惊悸,除邪气,明目开心益智。久服轻身延年(《本经》)。	[Indications] It is good for replenishing the Five Viscera (Liver, Heart, Spleen, Lung and Kidney), tranquilizing the spirit and pacifying the soul, relieving convulsions and palpitations, and dispersing pathogenic factors. It improves the eyesight and the intelligence. Long-term taking of the drug makes the patient happy and able to enjoy a long life. Shen Nong Bencao Jing (*Shennong's Great Herbal*)
疗肠胃中冷,心腹鼓痛,胸胁逆满,霍乱吐逆,调中,止消渴,通血脉,破坚积,令人不忘(《别录》)。	It warms a cold feeling in the stomach and intestines, and relieves pain and distention in the epigastrium and abdomen, and fullness and uneasiness in the chest and costal regions. It treats cholera with vomiting and adverse ascension of gas. It harmonizes the interior, quenches thirst in cases of diabetes, facilitates the blood circulation, and dissolves hardness and stagnation. It also strengthens the power of memory. Mingyi Bielu (*Records of Famous Doctors*)
主五劳七伤,虚损痰弱,止呕哕,补五脏六腑,保中守神。消胸中痰,治肺痿及痫疾,冷气逆上,伤寒不下食,凡虚而多梦纷纭者加之(甄权)。	Zhen Quan: It is good for treating five types of overstrain and seven types of injuries, consumptive diseases in persons of weak build and phlegm accumulation. It stops vomiting and nausea. It replenishes the Five Viscera (Liver, Heart, Spleen, Stomach, Large Intestine, Small Intestine, Urinary Bladder and Sanjiao), protects the interior and pacifies the mind. It eliminates phlegm from the thorax. It treats pulmonary flaccidity syndrome and epilepsy. It brings down adverse ascension of cold gas. It improves the appetite of a patient suffering from anorexia in case of a febrile disease caused by Cold. In treating a patient with deficient condition with dreamy sleep, Renshen/radix ginseng/ginseng root should be added to the prescription.

continued

原　文	罗希文译本
止烦躁,变酸水(李)。	Li Xun: It relieves restlessness and irritation, and reduces acid regurgitation.
消食开胃,调中治气,杀金石药毒(大明)。	Da Ming: It relieves indigestion and whets the appetite, harmonizes the interior and regulates the Vital Energy, and neutralizes the toxin in metal and stone drugs.
治肺胃阳气不足,肺气虚促,短气少气,补中缓中,泻心、肺、脾、胃中火邪,止渴生津液(元素)。	It replenishes the Yang Vital Energy in the Lung and Stomach. It treats shortness of breath due to deficient condition of the Lung. It replenishes and harmonizes the interior. It purges pathogenic Fire from the Heart, Lung, Spleen and Stomach. It quenches thirst and helps produce body fluid.
治男妇一切虚证,发热自汗,眩晕头痛,反胃吐食,疟,滑泻久痢,小便频数淋沥,劳倦内伤,中风中暑,瘦痹,吐血、嗽血、下血,血淋、血崩,胎前、产后诸病(时珍)。	It treats consumptive and deficient diseases of all kinds in both men and women, accompanied by fever and spontaneous perspiration, vertigo and headache, regurgitation and vomiting of food, pertinacious malaria, slippery diarrhea and dysentery, frequent urination and urinary dripping, consumptive disease with internal damage, heat stroke and invasion of pathogenic Wind, paralysis, hematemesis, coughing with blood and hematuria, stranguria with hematuria and metrorrhagia, and antepartum and postpartum diseases.

罗希文. 汉英对照 本草纲目选 [M].北京：外文出版社,2012：46-85.

Appendix Ⅱ English for TCM Subjects and Professionals

学科、专业人员名称中英文对照示例
Subjects and Professionals

序号	中 文 名 称	参 考 英 文
	学科	Subjects
1	中医学	Chinese medicine; traditional Chinese medicine (TCM)
2	中医基础理论	basic theory of Chinese medicine
3	中医诊断学	diagnostics of Chinese medicine
4	中医内科学	Chinese internal medicine
5	中医外科学	Chinese external medicine; surgery of Chinese medicine
6	中医妇科学	Chinese gynecology; gynecology of Chinese medicine
7	中医儿科学	Chinese pediatrics; pediatrics of Chinese medicine
8	中医骨伤科学	Chinese orthopedics and traumatology; orthopedics and traumatology of Chinese medicine
9	正骨	Bonesetting; ulna
10	中医眼科学	Chinese ophthalmology; ophthalmology of Chinese medicine
11	中医耳鼻喉科学	Chinese otorhinolaryngology; otorhinolaryngology of Chinese medicine
12	中医皮肤病学	Chinese dermatology; dermatology of Chinese medicine
13	中医肛肠病学	Chinese proctology; proctology of Chinese medicine
14	中医急诊学	Chinese emergency medicine
15	针灸学	acupuncture and moxibustion
16	经络学	meridian/channel and collateral
17	腧穴学	acupuncture points
18	刺法灸法学	acupuncture and moxibustion technique
19	针灸治疗学	acupuncture and moxibustion therapy
20	实验针灸学	experimental acupuncture and moxibustion
21	推拿学	tuina
22	推拿手法学	manipulation of tuina
23	针刀医学	acupotomy
24	中医养生学	Chinese health preservation

continued

序号	中 文 名 称	参 考 英 文
25	中医康复学	rehabilitation of Chinese medicine
26	中医食疗学	diet therapy of Chinese medicine
27	中医药膳学	medicated diet of Chinese medicine
28	中医护理学	Chinese nursing
29	十三科	thirteen branches of medicine
30	中药学	Chinese materia medica; Chinese pharmacy
31	本草	materia medica
32	本草学	material medica
33	方剂学	Chinese medical formulas
34	中草药	Chinese herbal medicine
35	中成药学	Chinese patent medicine
36	药用植物学	pharmaceutical botany
37	中药化学	Chinese medicinal chemistry
38	中药药理学	Chinese pharmacology; pharmacology of Chinese medicine
39	中药鉴别学	Chinese medicinal identification
40	中药炮制学	Chinese medicinal processing
41	中药药剂学	Chinese pharmaceutics; pharmaceutics of Chinese medicine
42	中药制剂分析	analysis of Chinese pharmaceutical preparation
43	中医医史学	history of Chinese medicine
44	中医文献学	Chinese medical literature
45	中医各家学说	various schools of traditional Chinese medicine
46	医古文	medical articles of archaic Chinese
47	中医医案	case records of Chinese medicine
48	黄帝内经	Huangdi's Internal Classic
49	素问	Plain Questions
50	灵枢	Miraculous Pivot
51	内经	Internal Classic
52	金匮要略	Synopsis of the Golden Chamber
53	伤寒论	Treatise on Cold Damage Diseases
54	温病学	warm diseases
55	中西医结合	integration of Chinese and Western medicine
	专业人员	**Professionals**
56	中医	Chinese medicine; physician/doctor of Chinese medicine
57	中医师	physician/doctor of Chinese medicine
58	中药师	pharmacist of Chinese medicine

continued

序号	中 文 名 称	参 考 英 文
59	针灸师	acupuncturist
60	推拿按摩师	massagist
61	中西医结合医师	physician/doctor of integrated Chinese and Western medicine
62	中医护士	nurse of Chinese medicine
63	草药医生	herbalist
64	疡医	sore and wound doctor

源自世界中医药学会联合会（World Federation of Chinese Medicine Societies）2007 年发布的《中医基本名词术语中英对照国际标准》（*International Standard Chinese-English Basic Nomenclature of Chinese Medicine*）。

Appendix Ⅲ Supplementary Chapter Traditional Medicine Conditions of ICD‑11

国际疾病分类第 11 版(ICD‑11)传统医学章节(中英对照表)

序号	中　文	英　文	Inclusions/Exclusions
1	传统医学疾病	Traditional medicine disorders	
2	脏腑系统疾病	Organ system disorders	
3	肝系病类	Liver system disorders	
4	胁痛	Hypochondrium pain disorder	
5	黄疸	Jaundice disorder	Inclusions：Acute jaundice；Yang jaundice；Yin jaundice
6	肝著	Liver distension disorder	
7	鼓胀	Tympanites disorder	Inclusions：Tympanism disorder；Tympany disorder
8	肝痈	Liver abscess disorder	
9	胆胀	Gallbladder distension disorder	
10	其他特指的肝系病类	Other specified liver system disorders	
11	未特指的肝系病类	Liver system disorders, unspecified	
12	心系病类	Heart system disorders	
13	心悸	Palpitation disorders	
14	惊悸	Inducible palpitation disorder	Inclusions：Fright palpitation disorder
15	怔忡	Spontaneous palpitation disorder	Inclusions：Fearful throbbing disorder
16	其他特指的心悸	Other specified palpitation disorders	
17	未特指的心悸	Palpitation disorders, unspecified	
18	胸痹	Chest impediment disorders	Inclusions：Heart pain disorder；Chest impediment disorder
19	真心痛	True heart pain disorder	Inclusions：Severe heart pain disorder
20	其他特指的胸痹	Other specified chest impediment disorders	
21	未特指的胸痹	Chest impediment disorders, unspecified	
22	其他特指的心系病类	Other specified heart system disorders	

continued

序号	中　文	英　文	Inclusions/Exclusions
23	未特指的心系病类	Heart system disorders, unspecified	
24	脾系病类	Spleen system disorders	
25	噎膈	Dysphagia disorder	Inclusions：Choke disorder
26	胃脘痛	Stomach ache disorder	
27	胃胀	Epigastric distension disorder	
28	嘈杂	Epigastric upset disorder	
29	食积	Food retention disorder	Inclusions： Food accumulation disorder
30	泄泻	Diarrhea disorder	
31	痢疾	Dysentery disorder	
32	便秘	Constipation disorder	
33	腹痛	Abdominal pain disorder	Exclusions： Lower abdominal colic disorder
34	肠痈	Intestinal abscess disorder	
35	其他特指的脾系病类	Other specified spleen system disorders	
36	未特指的脾系病类	Spleen system disorders, unspecified	
37	肺系病类	Lung system disorders	
38	感冒	Common cold disorder	Exclusions： Seasonal cold disorder
39	咳嗽	Cough disorders	
40	咳逆	Cough with dyspnea disorder	Exclusions：Panting disorder； Dyspnea disorder
41	其他特指的咳嗽	Other specified cough disorders	
42	未特指的咳嗽	Cough disorders, unspecified	
43	喘证	Dyspnea disorder	Inclusions：Panting disorder Exclusions： Cough with dyspnea disorder
44	哮病	Wheezing disorder	
45	肺胀	Lung distension disorder	
46	悬饮	Pleural fluid retention disorder	
47	肺热病	Lung heat disorder	
48	肺痿	Lung withering disorder	
49	结胸	Chest bind disorder	
50	其他特指的肺系病类	Other specified lung system disorders	
51	未特指的肺系病类	Lung system disorders, unspecified	
52	肾系病类	Kidney system disorders	
53	淋证	Strangury disorders	

continued

序号	中　文	英　文	Inclusions/Exclusions
54	石淋	Stony stranguria disorder	
55	热淋	Heat stranguria disorder	
56	其他特指的淋证	Other specified strangury disorders	
57	未特指的淋证	Strangury disorders, unspecified	
58	肾著	Kidney stagnation disorder	
59	尿崩	Flooding urine disorder	
60	遗尿	Enuresis disorder	
61	尿浊	Turbid urine disorder	
62	癃闭	Dribbling urinary block disorder	Inclusions：Ischuria disorder
63	关格	Block and repulsion disorder	Inclusions：Dysuria and frequent vomiting disorder
64	水肿	Edema disorders	
65	肾水	Kidney edema disorder	
66	风水	Wind edema disorder	
67	其他特指的水肿	Other specified edema disorders	
68	未特指的水肿	Edema disorders, unspecified	
69	疝气	Lower abdominal colic disorder	Inclusions：Hernia Exclusions：Abdominal pain disorder
70	早泄	Premature ejaculation disorder	
71	遗精	Involuntary ejaculation disorder	
72	阳强	Persistent erection disorder	
73	阳痿	Impotence disorder	
74	不育	Male Infertility disorder	Inclusions： Male Sterility disorder
75	其他特指的肾系病类	Other specified kidney system disorders	
76	未特指的肾系病类	Kidney system disorders, unspecified	
77	其他特指的脏腑系统疾病	Other specified organ system disorders	
78	未特指的脏腑系统疾病	Organ system disorders, unspecified	
79	其他身体系统疾病	Other body system disorders	
80	皮肤黏膜系统病类	Skin and mucosa system disorders	
81	湿疮	Dampness sore disorder	Inclusions：Eczema disorder
82	黄水疮	Impetigo disorder	
83	疔疮	Furuncle disorders	Inclusions：Boil disorders
84	疔疮走黄	Septicemic furunculosis disorder	
85	其他特指的疔疮	Other specified furuncle disorders	

continued

序号	中　文	英　文	Inclusions/Exclusions
86	未特指的疔疮	Furuncle disorders, unspecified	
87	褥疮	Bed sore disorder	Inclusions：Decubitus disorder
88	痈证	Abscess disorders	
89	流注	Deep multiple abscess disorder	Inclusions：Multiple abscesses disorder
90	肛痈	Anal abscess disorder	
91	其他特指的痈证	Other specified abscess disorders	
92	未特指的痈证	Abscess disorders, unspecified	
93	疽证	Headed carbuncle disorder	
94	脚湿气	Foot dampness itch disorder	Inclusions：Smelly snail disorder
95	圆癣	Tinea circinate disorder	Inclusions：Tinea corporis disorder
96	蛇皮癣	Dry skin disorder	Inclusions：Ichthyosis disorder
97	脱疽	Gangrene disorder	Inclusions：Toe gangrene disorder
98	疣	Wart disorder	
99	鹅掌风	Hand dampness itch disorder	Inclusions：Goose web wind disorder
100	丹毒	Erysipelas disorder	
101	发证	Cellulitis disorder	
102	鹅口疮	Thrush disorder	
103	蛇串疮	Herpes zoster disorder	Inclusions：Herpes zoster around the waist and hypochondrium disorder；Snake-shaped herpes zoster, herpes zoster around the waist and hypochondria；Snake-clustered sores disorder
104	内痔	Interior haemorroid disorder	
105	肛裂	Fissured anus disorder	
106	其他特指的皮肤黏膜系统病类	Other specified skin and mucosa system disorders	
107	未特指的皮肤黏膜系统病类	Skin and mucosa system disorders, unspecified	
108	女性生殖系统(包括分娩)病类	Female reproductive system disorders (including childbirth)	
109	月经病类	Menstruation associated disorders	
110	月经周期病	Menstruation cycle disorders	Inclusions：Menstrual cycle disorders

continued

序号	中　文	英　文	Inclusions/Exclusions
111	月经先期	Advanced menstruation disorder	
112	月经后期	Delayed menstruation disorder	
113	月经先后无定期	Irregular menstruation disorders	
114	其他特指的月经周期病	Other specified menstruation cycle disorders	
115	未特指的月经周期病	Menstruation cycle disorders, unspecified	
116	月经过多	Menorrhagia disorder	Inclusions：Hypermenorrhea disorder
117	月经过少	Decreased menstruation disorder	Inclusions：Scanty menstruation disorder
118	经期延长	Prolonged menstruation disorder	
119	崩漏	Metrorrhagia disorder	
120	闭经	Amenorrhea disorder	Inclusions：No periods disorder
121	绝经前后诸症	Menopausal disorder	
122	痛经	Dysmenorrhea disorder	Inclusions：Menstrual cramp disorder；Painful periods disorder
123	其他特指的月经病类	Other specified menstruation associated disorders	
124	未特指的月经病类	Menstruation associated disorders, unspecified	
125	妊娠病类	Pregnancy associated disorders	
126	恶阻	Morning sickness disorder	Inclusions：Vomiting during pregnancy disorder
127	胎动不安	Unstable fetus disorder	
128	转胞	Bladder pressure disorder	Inclusions：Shifted colic disorder；Shifted bladder disorder；Bladder colic disorder
129	子痫	Eclampsia disorder	
130	子悬	Floating sensation pregnancy disorder	Inclusions：Gravid oppression disorder；Pregnancy suspension disorder
131	其他特指的妊娠病类	Other specified pregnancy associated disorders	
132	未特指的妊娠病类	Pregnancy associated disorders, unspecified	
133	产后病类	Puerperium associated disorders	
134	儿枕痛	Puerperal abdominal pain disorder	Inclusions：Postpartum abdominal pain disorder
135	产后风	Puerperal wind disorder	Inclusions：Convulsions after childbirth disorder；Postpartum spasm disorder

continued

序号	中 文	英 文	Inclusions/Exclusions
136	缺乳	Hypogalactia disorder	
137	恶露不绝	Postpartum lochiorrhea disorder	
138	其他特指的产后病类	Other specified puerperium associated disorders	
139	未特指的产后病类	Puerperium associated disorders, unspecified	
140	其他女性生殖系统病类	Other female reproductive system associated disorders	
141	带下病	Leukorrhea disorder	Inclusions： Vaginal discharge disorder
142	阴吹	Vaginal flatus disorder	
143	不孕	Infertility disorder	Inclusions： Female infertility disorder； Female sterility disorder Exclusions： Male Infertility disorder
144	石瘕	Uterine mass disorder	Inclusions： Stony womb mass disorder
145	乳癖	Breast lump disorder	Inclusions：Hyperplasia of mammary gland disorder； Fibrocystic breast disorder
146	其他特指的其他女性生殖系统病类	Other specified other female reproductive system associated disorders	
147	未特指的其他女性生殖系统病类	Other female reproductive system associated disorders, unspecified	
148	其他特指的女性生殖系统（包括分娩）病类	Other specified female reproductive system disorders (including childbirth)	
149	未特指的女性生殖系统(包括分娩)病类	Female reproductive system disorders (including childbirth), unspecified	
150	骨、关节和肌肉系统病类	Bone, joint and muscle system disorders	
151	痹病	Joint impediment disorders	Inclusions：Impediment disorders；Hindrance disorders
152	痛痹	Cold impediment disorder	Inclusions： Cold hindrance disorder； Painful impediment disorder
153	行痹	Wind impediment disorder	Inclusions：Moving impediment disorder；Wind hindrance disorder；Migrating painful movement disorder；Migratory impediment
154	着痹	Dampness impediment disorder	Inclusions： Dampness hindrance disorder； Fixed impediment disorder

continued

序号	中　文	英　文	Inclusions/Exclusions
155	其他特指的痹病	Other specified joint impediment disorders	
156	未特指的痹病	Joint impediment disorders, unspecified	
157	转筋	Muscle spasm disorder	Inclusions: Muscle cramp disorder
158	腰痛	Lumbago disorder	Inclusions: Low back pain disorder
159	麻木	Numbness disorder	
160	痿证	Wilting disorder	
161	其他特指的骨、关节和肌肉系统病类	Other specified bone, joint and muscle system disorders	
162	未特指的骨、关节和肌肉系统病类	Bone, joint and muscle system disorders, unspecified	
163	眼、耳、鼻和喉系统病类	Eye, ear, nose and throat system disorders	
164	高风内障[雀目]	Night blindness disorder	Inclusions: Nyctalopia disorder
165	五风内障	Wind glaucoma disorder	
166	胞肿如桃	Inflammatory eyelid disorder	
167	胞虚如球	Non-inflammatory eyelid disorder	
168	混睛障	Corneal opacity disorder	
169	耳鸣	Tinnitus disorder	Exclusions: Cerebral tinnitus disorder
170	耳聋	Deafness disorders	
171	暴聋	Sudden deafness disorder	
172	渐聋	Gradual deafness disorder	
173	其他特指的耳聋	Other specified deafness disorders	
174	未特指的耳聋	Deafness disorders, unspecified	
175	鼻鼽	Allergic rhinitis disorder	
176	鼻渊	Nasal sinusitis disorder	
177	喉喑	Hoarseness disorder	
178	乳蛾	Tonsillitis disorder	
179	其他特指的眼、耳、鼻和喉系统病类	Other specified eye, ear, nose and throat system disorders	
180	未特指的眼、耳、鼻和喉系统病类	Eye, ear, nose and throat system disorders, unspecified	
181	脑系病类	Brain system disorders	
182	口僻	Facial paralysis disorder	Inclusions: Wry mouth disorder
183	头痛	Headache disorders	
184	偏头风	Migraine disorder	Inclusions: Migraine pain disorder

continued

序号	中　文	英　文	Inclusions/Exclusions
185	头风	Head wind disorder	
186	其他特指的头痛	Other specified headache disorders	
187	未特指的头痛	Headache disorders, unspecified	
188	痉痓	Convulsion disorder	Inclusions：Convulsive disorder；Postpartum convulsion disorder
189	脑鸣	Cerebral tinnitus disorder	Exclusions：Tinnitus disorder
190	眩晕	Vertigo disorder	
191	健忘	Forgetfulness disorder	
192	弄舌	Frequent protrusion of tongue disorder	
193	中风	Wind stroke disorders	
194	中风先兆证	Prodrome of wind stroke disorder	Inclusions：Onset of wind stroke Exclusions：Sequela of wind stroke disorder
195	中风后遗证	Sequela of wind stroke disorder	Exclusions：Prodrome of wind stroke disorder
196	其他特指的中风	Other specified wind stroke disorders	
197	未特指的中风	Wind stroke disorders, unspecified	
198	厥症	Syncope disorder	Inclusions：Qi syncope disorder；Blood syncope disorder；Phlegm syncope disorder；Hunger syncope disorder；Cold syncope disorder Exclusions：wasting thirst related syncope disorder
199	其他特指的脑系病类	Other specified brain system disorders	
200	未特指的脑系病类	Brain system disorders, unspecified	
201	其他特指的其他身体系统疾病	Other specified other body system disorders	
202	未特指的其他身体系统疾病	Other body system disorders, unspecified	
203	气血津液病	Qi, blood and fluid disorders	
204	气瘿	Qi goiter disorder	
205	消渴	Wasting thirst disorder	
206	虚劳	Consumptive disorder	
207	其他特指的气血津液病	Other specified qi, blood and fluid disorders	
208	未特指的气血津液病	Qi, blood and fluid disorders, unspecified	
209	精神情志病类	Mental and emotional disorders	

continued

序号	中　文	英　文	Inclusions/Exclusions
210	百合病	Lily disorder	Exclusions：Hysteria disorder；Insomnia disorders
211	躁病	Manic disorder	
212	郁证	Depression disorder	Inclusions：Melancholy disorder；Depressive disorder；Postpartum depression disorder；Pregnancy depression disorder
213	脏躁	Uneasiness disorder	Exclusions：Depression disorder；Lily disorder
214	不寐	Insomnia disorder	
215	多寐	Somnolence disorder	
216	痴呆	Dementia disorder	Inclusions：Aged dementia disorders Exclusions：Amnesia disorder
217	火病	Repressed fire disorder	Inclusions：Fire disorder；Repressed anger disorder
218	其他特指的精神情志病类	Other specified mental and emotional disorders	
219	未特指的精神情志病类	Mental and emotional disorders, unspecified	
220	外感病	External contraction disorders	
221	时行感冒	Seasonal cold disorder	Exclusions：Common cold disorder
222	劳瘵	Fatigue consumption disorder	Exclusions：Flowing phlegm disorder
223	霍乱	Severe vomiting and diarrhoea disorder	Exclusions：Diarrhea disorder；Cholera
224	疟疾	Alternating fever and chills disorder	Exclusions：Malaria
225	蛊病	Parasitic disorder	
226	流痰	Flowing phlegm disorder	Inclusions：Bone and joint tuberculosis disorder
227	温病	Warmth disorders	
228	暑温	Summer-heat disorder	
229	春温	Spring warmth disorder	
230	湿温	Dampness and warmth disorder	
231	其他特指的温病	Other specified warmth disorders	
232	未特指的温病	Warmth disorders, unspecified	
233	其他特指的外感病	Other specified external contraction disorders	
234	未特指的外感病	External contraction disorders, unspecified	

continued

序号	中　文	英　文	Inclusions/Exclusions
235	儿童期与青少年期病类	Childhood and adolescence associated disorders	
236	迟证	Developmental delay disorder	
237	变蒸热	Growth fever disorder	
238	生长痛	Growth pain disorder	
239	急惊风	Acute convulsion disorder	
240	慢惊风	Recurrent convulsion disorder	
241	客忤	Fright seizure disorder	
242	夜啼	Night crying disorder	
243	疳病	Infantile malnutrition disorder	
244	滞遗	Dribbling disorder	
245	臀红	Diaper dermatitis disorder	
246	硬证	Infant stiffness disorder	
247	软证	Infant limpness disorder	Inclusions：Infant flaccidity disorder；Infant flaccid disorder
248	其他特指的儿童期与青少年期病类	Other specified childhood and adolescence associated disorders	
249	未特指的儿童期与青少年期病类	Childhood and adolescence associated disorders, unspecified	
250	其他特指的传统医学疾病	Other specified traditional medicine disorders	
251	未特指的传统医学疾病	Traditional medicine disorders, unspecified	
252	传统医学证候	Traditional medicine patterns	
253	八纲证	Principle-based patterns	
254	阳证	Yang pattern	
255	阴证	Yin pattern	
256	热证	Heat pattern	
257	寒证	Cold pattern	
258	实证	Excess pattern	
259	虚证	Deficiency pattern	
260	表证	Exterior pattern	
261	里证	Interior pattern	
262	寒热中间证	Moderate (Heat/Cold) pattern	
263	虚实中间证	Medium (Excess/Deficiency) pattern	
264	寒热错杂证	Tangled cold and heat pattern	
265	其他特指的八纲证	Other specified principle-based patterns	

continued

序号	中　　文	英　　文	Inclusions/Exclusions
266	未特指的八纲证	Principle-based patterns, unspecified	
267	外感证	Environmental factor patterns	
268	风淫证	Wind factor pattern	
269	寒淫证	Cold factor pattern	
270	湿淫证	Dampness factor pattern	
271	燥淫证	Dryness factor pattern	
272	火热淫证	Fire-heat factor pattern	
273	暑淫证	Summer-heat factor pattern	
274	疫疠证	Pestilent factor pattern	
275	其他特指的外感证	Other specified environmental factor patterns	
276	未特指的外感证	Environmental factor patterns, unspecified	
277	气血津液证	Body constituents patterns	
278	气证	Qi patterns	Exclusions：Qi phase patterns
279	气虚证	Qi deficiency pattern	Inclusions：Qi decrease pattern
280	气滞证	Qi stagnation pattern	Inclusions：Qi depression pattern
281	气逆证	Qi uprising pattern	Inclusions：Qi reflux pattern; Qi counterflow pattern; Qi rising pattern
282	气陷证	Qi sinking pattern	Inclusions：Qi fall pattern
283	气脱证	Qi collapse pattern	Inclusions：Primordial qi collapse pattern
284	其他特指的气证	Other specified qi patterns	
285	未特指的气证	Qi patterns, unspecified	
286	血证	Blood patterns	Exclusions：Blood phase patterns
287	血虚证	Blood deficiency pattern	Inclusions：Blood decrease patterns
288	血瘀证	Blood stasis pattern	Inclusions：Blood stagnation pattern
289	血热证	Blood heat pattern	Exclusions：Blood cold pattern
290	血寒证	Blood cold pattern	Exclusions：Qi patterns; Blood heat pattern
291	血燥证	Blood dryness pattern	Exclusions：Qi patterns; Blood heat pattern
292	其他特指的血证	Other specified blood patterns	
293	未特指的血证	Blood patterns, unspecified	
294	津液证	Fluid patterns（BlockL3-SF1）	

continued

序号	中　文	英　文	Inclusions/Exclusions
295	津液亏虚证	Fluid deficiency pattern	Inclusions： Fluid decrease pattern Exclusions： Essence deficiency pattern
296	水毒证	Fluid disturbance pattern	Inclusions： Fluid dysfunction pattern；Fluid retention pattern
297	燥痰证	Dry-phlegm pattern	
298	湿痰证	Damp phlegm pattern	
299	痰火扰心证	Phlegm-fire harassing the heart system pattern	
300	风痰证	Wind-phlegm pattern	
301	其他特指的津液证	Other specified fluid patterns	
302	未特指的津液证	Fluid patterns, unspecified	
303	精证	Essence patterns	
304	精虚证	Essence deficiency pattern	
305	其他特指的精证	Other specified essence patterns	
306	未特指的精证	Essence patterns, unspecified	
307	其他特指的气血津液证	Other specified body constituents patterns	
308	未特指的气血津液证	Body constituents patterns, unspecified	
309	脏腑证	Organ system patterns	
310	肝系证类	Liver system patterns	
311	肝阴虚证	Liver yin deficiency pattern	Inclusions： Liver deficiency-heat pattern
312	肝阳虚证	Liver yang deficiency pattern	Inclusions： Liver deficiency-cold pattern
313	肝阳上亢证	Liver yang ascendant hyperactivity pattern	
314	肝气虚证	Liver qi deficiency pattern	
315	肝血虚证	Liver blood deficiency pattern	
316	肝郁血瘀证	Liver depression and blood stasis pattern	Inclusions： Pattern of liver blood stasis and stagnation；Pattern of liver stasis with qi stagnation
317	肝风内动证	Liver wind stirring the interior pattern	Inclusions： Internal stirring of liver wind
318	肝气化火证	Liver qi stagnation pattern	Inclusions： Liver meridian stagnated heat pattern；Liver depression and qi stagnation pattern
319	肝火上炎证	Liver fire flaming upward pattern	Inclusions：Hyperactivity of liver fire pattern

continued

序号	中　文	英　文	Inclusions/Exclusions
320	肝热动风证	Liver heat stirring wind pattern	Inclusions：Pattern of heat stirring liver wind
321	肝胆湿热证	Liver-gallbladder dampness-heat pattern	Inclusions：Damp-heat in liver-gallbladder
322	肝经湿热证	Liver meridian dampness-heat pattern	
323	寒滞肝脉证	Liver meridian cold stagnation pattern	Inclusions：Cold stagnation in liver meridian pattern；Liver meridian excess cold pattern；Liver cold pattern
324	胆气虚证	Gallbladder qi deficiency pattern	Inclusions：Gallbladder insufficiency with timidity；Gallbladder deficiency with qi timidity
325	胆郁痰扰证	Gallbladder depression with phlegm harassment pattern	Inclusions：Stagnation of gallbladder and disturbance of phlegm pattern
326	胆热证	Gallbladder heat pattern	Inclusions：Gallbladder meridian depressed heat pattern；Heat stagnation in the gallbladder meridian pattern；Gallbladder fire pattern
327	胆寒证	Gallbladder cold pattern	
328	肝肾阴虚证	Liver and kidney yin deficiency pattern	
329	肝脾不和证	Disharmony of liver and spleen systems pattern	Inclusions：Liver depression and spleen deficiency pattern；Imbalance between liver and spleen pattern
330	肝胃不和证	Disharmony of liver and stomach systems pattern	Inclusions：Liver qi invading the stomach pattern；Liver-stomach disharmony pattern；Disharmony between liver and stomach pattern
331	肝火犯胃证	Liver fire invading the stomach system pattern	
332	肝火犯肺证	Liver fire invading the lung system pattern	Inclusions：Wood fire tormenting metal pattern
333	其他特指的肝系证类	Other specified liver system patterns	
334	未特指的肝系证类	Liver system patterns, unspecified	
335	心系证类	Heart system patterns	
336	心气虚证	Heart qi deficiency pattern	
337	心血虚证	Heart blood deficiency pattern	

continued

序号	中　文	英　文	Inclusions/Exclusions
338	心气血两虚证	Dual deficiency of heart qi and blood pattern	
339	心脉痹阻证	Heart meridian obstruction pattern	
340	心阴虚证	Heart yin deficiency pattern	Inclusions：Heart yin depletion pattern
341	心气阴两虚证	Deficiency of heart qi and yin pattern	
342	心阳虚证	Heart yang deficiency pattern	
343	心阳暴脱证	Heart yang collapse pattern	
344	心火上炎证	Heart fire flaming upward pattern	
345	热扰心神证	Fire harassing heart spirit pattern	
346	水气凌心证	Water qi intimidating the heart system pattern	
347	心神不宁证	Heart spirit restlessness pattern	
348	忧伤神气证	Anxiety damaging the spirit pattern	Inclusions：Pattern of melancholy damaging spirit
349	小肠气滞证	Small intestine qi stagnation pattern	
350	小肠实热证	Small intestine excess heat pattern	
351	小肠虚寒证	Small intestine deficiency cold pattern	
352	心肝血虚证	Heart and liver blood deficiency pattern	
353	心胆气虚证	Heart and gallbladder qi deficiency pattern	
354	心脾两虚证	Heart and spleen systems deficiency pattern	
355	心肺气虚证	Heart and lung qi deficiency pattern	
356	心肾不交证	Heart and kidney systems disharmony pattern	
357	心肾阳虚证	Heart and kidney yang deficiency pattern	
358	其他特指的心系证类	Other specified heart system patterns	
359	未特指的心系证类	Heart system patterns, unspecified	
360	脾系证类	Spleen system patterns	
361	脾气虚证	Spleen qi deficiency pattern	Inclusions：Spleen qi depletion pattern
362	脾气下陷证	Spleen qi sinking pattern	Inclusions：Middle qi sinking pattern
363	脾虚气滞证	Spleen deficiency with qi stagnation pattern	
364	脾虚食积证	Spleen deficiency with food retention pattern	
365	脾不统血证	Spleen failing to control the blood pattern	
366	脾虚血亏证	Spleen deficiency and blood depletion pattern	

continued

序号	中　文	英　文	Inclusions/Exclusions
367	脾阴虚证	Spleen yin deficiency pattern	Inclusions： Spleen yin depletion pattern
368	脾阳虚证	Spleen yang depletion pattern	Inclusions：Pattern of spleen deficiency and cold；Spleen yang depletion pattern
369	湿热蕴脾证	Dampness-heat encumbering the spleen system pattern	Inclusions：Damp heat in the spleen system pattern；Dampness and heat in the spleen and stomach systems pattern；Dampness encumbering the spleen and stomach systems pattern
370	脾虚湿困证	Spleen deficiency with dampness accumulation pattern	Inclusions：Spleen deficiency with dampness encumbrance pattern
371	脾虚水泛证	Spleen deficiency with water flooding pattern	Inclusions：Spleen qi deficiency with water retention pattern；Spleen qi deficiency with dampness pattern
372	寒湿困脾证	Cold-dampness encumbering the spleen system pattern	
373	胃气虚证	Stomach qi deficiency pattern	
374	胃气上逆证	Stomach qi uprising pattern	Inclusions：Stomach qi reverse flow pattern
375	胃阴虚证	Stomach yin deficiency pattern	Inclusions：Stomach yin depletion pattern；Stomach deficiency and heat pattern
376	胃热证	Stomach heat pattern	
377	湿阻肠道证	Dampness in the intestines pattern	
378	寒邪犯胃证	Cold invading the stomach system pattern	Inclusions： Stomach cold excess pattern
379	寒滞肠道证	Intestine cold stagnation pattern	
380	思伤脾气证	Anxiety damaging the spleen system pattern	
381	肺脾两虚证	Lung and spleen deficiency pattern	
382	脾肾阳虚证	Spleen and kidney yang deficiency pattern	
383	其他特指的脾系证类	Other specified spleen system patterns	
384	未特指的脾系证类	Spleen system patterns, unspecified	
385	肺病证类	Lung system patterns	
386	肺气虚证	Lung qi deficiency pattern	
387	肺阴虚证	Lung yin deficiency pattern	
388	肺肾阴虚证	Lung and kidney yin deficiency pattern	

continued

序号	中　文	英　文	Inclusions/Exclusions
389	肺气阴两虚证	Lung qi and yin deficiency pattern	
390	肺阳虚证	Lung yang deficiency pattern	
391	寒痰阻肺证	Cold phlegm obstructing the lung pattern	
392	痰浊阻肺证	Turbid phlegm accumulation in the lung pattern	
393	表寒肺热证	Exterior cold with lung heat pattern	
394	肺热炽盛证	Intense congestion of lung heat pattern	Inclusions： Intense lung heat pattern
395	痰热壅肺证	Phlegm heat obstructing the lung pattern	
396	风热犯肺证	Wind-heat invading the lung pattern	
397	肺热移肠证	Lung heat transmitting into the intestine pattern	
398	风寒束肺证	Wind-cold fettering the lung pattern	
399	燥邪犯肺证	Dryness invading the lung pattern	
400	肺燥肠闭证	Lung dryness with intestinal obstruction pattern	
401	大肠实热证	Large intestine excess heat pattern	
402	大肠湿热证	Large intestine dampness heat pattern	
403	大肠津亏证	Large intestine fluid deficiency pattern	
404	大肠虚寒证	Large intestine deficiency cold pattern	
405	其他特指的肺系证类	Other specified lung system patterns	
406	未特指的肺系证类	Lung system patterns, unspecified	
407	肾病证类	Kidney system patterns	
408	肾气虚证	Kidney qi deficiency pattern	Inclusions： Kidney qi depletion pattern
409	肾不纳气证	Kidney failing to receive qi pattern	Inclusions：Lung-kidney deficiency pattern；Insufficient qi of the lung and kidney pattern
410	肾气虚水泛证	Kidney qi deficiency with water retention pattern	Inclusions：Kidney qi deficiency with water flooding pattern
411	肾阴虚证	Kidney yin deficiency pattern	Inclusions：Genuine yin deficiency pattern；Kidney water depletion and deficiency pattern； Primordial yin deficiency pattern
412	肾阴阳两虚证	Kidney yin and yang deficiency pattern	
413	肾虚髓亏证	Kidney deficiency with marrow depletion pattern	

continued

序号	中　文	英　文	Inclusions/Exclusions
414	肾精亏虚证	Kidney essence deficiency pattern	
415	肾阳虚证	Kidney yang deficiency pattern	Inclusions：Life-gate fire depletion pattern；Primordial yang deficiency pattern
416	惊恐伤肾证	Fear damaging the kidney system pattern	
417	胞宫血热证	Blood and heat accumulation in the uterus pattern	Inclusions：Blood heat build up in the uterus pattern
418	痰凝胞宫证	Phlegm obstructing the uterus pattern	Inclusions：Phlegm congealment in the uterus pattern；Dampness Phlegm obstructing the uterus pattern
419	胞宫湿热证	Dampness-heat in the uterus pattern	
420	寒凝胞宫证	Cold stagnation in the uterus pattern	Inclusions：Cold congealment in the uterus pattern
421	胞宫虚寒证	Uterine deficiency cold pattern	Inclusions：Uterine yang deficiency pattern
422	膀胱蓄血证	Blood accumulation in the bladder pattern	Inclusions：Blood and heat build up in the bladder pattern
423	膀胱蕴热证	Bladder heat accumulation pattern	Inclusions：Bladder heat retention pattern；Bladder heat excess pattern
424	膀胱湿热证	Bladder dampness-heat pattern	
425	膀胱蓄水证	Bladder water accumulation pattern	Inclusions：Water amassment in the bladder pattern
426	膀胱虚寒证	Bladder deficiency cold pattern	
427	其他特指的肾系证类	Other specified kidney system patterns	
428	未特指的肾系证类	Kidney system patterns, unspecified	
429	其他特指的脏腑证类	Other specified organ system patterns	
430	未特指的脏腑证类	Organ system patterns, unspecified	
431	经络证	Meridian and collateral patterns	
432	十二正经证	Main Meridian Patterns	
433	手太阴肺经 是动病证	Lung meridian pattern	
434	手阳明大肠经 是动病证	Large intestine meridian pattern	
435	足阳明胃经 是动病证	Stomach meridian pattern	
436	足太阴脾经 是动病证	Spleen meridian pattern	
437	手少阴心经 是动病证	Heart meridian pattern	
438	手太阳小肠经 是动病证	Small intestine meridian pattern	
439	足太阳膀胱经 是动病证	Bladder meridian pattern	
440	足少阴肾经 是动病证	Kidney meridian pattern	

continued

序号	中 文	英 文	Inclusions/Exclusions
441	手厥阴心包经 是动病证	Pericardium meridian pattern	Inclusions：Heart ruler meridian pattern；Heart governor meridian pattern
442	手少阳三焦经 是动病证	Triple energizer meridian pattern	Inclusions：Triple burner meridian pattern；Triple warmer meridian pattern
443	足少阳胆经 是动病证	Gallbladder meridian pattern	
444	足厥阴肝经 是动病证	Liver meridian pattern	
445	其他特指的十二正经证	Other specified main Meridian Patterns	
446	未特指的十二正经证	Main Meridian Patterns, unspecified	
447	奇经八脉证	Extra Meridian Patterns	
448	督脉病证	Governor vessel pattern	
449	任脉病证	Conception vessel pattern	
450	阴跷脉病证	Yin heel vessel pattern	
451	阳跷脉病证	Yang heel vessel pattern	
452	阴维脉病证	Yin link vessel pattern	
453	阳维脉病证	Yang link vessel pattern	
454	冲脉病证	Thoroughfare vessel pattern	
455	带脉病证	Belt vessel pattern	
456	其他特指的奇经八脉证	Other specified extra Meridian Patterns	
457	未特指的奇经八脉证	Extra Meridian Patterns, unspecified	
458	其他特指的经络证	Other specified meridian and collateral patterns	
459	未特指经络证的	Meridian and collateral patterns, unspecified	
460	六经证	Six stage patterns	Inclusions：Shanghan Patterns
461	太阳病证	Early yang stage pattern	Inclusions：Taiyang patterns；Greater yang pattern
462	阳明病证	Middle yang stage pattern	Inclusions：Yangming patterns；Yang brightness pattern
463	少阳病证	Late yang stage pattern	Inclusions：Shaoyang patterns；Lesser yang pattern
464	太阴病证	Early yin stage pattern	Inclusions：Taiyin patterns；Greater yin pattern
465	少阴病证	Middle yin stage Pattern, Middle yin stage pattern	Inclusions：Shaoyin Patterns；Lesser yin pattern
466	厥阴病证	Late Yin stage Patterns	Inclusions：Jueyin patterns；Reverting yin pattern
467	其他特指的六经证	Other specified six stage patterns	

continued

序号	中　文	英　文	Inclusions/Exclusions
468	未特指的六经证	Six stage patterns, unspecified	
469	三焦证	Triple energizer stage patterns	Inclusions：Wenbing Sanjiao Patterns；Triple Energizer Patterns；Triple Burner Patterns；Three Region Patterns
470	上焦证	Upper energizer stage patterns	Inclusions：Upper energizer patterns；Upper Burner Patterns；Upper Region Patterns
471	中焦证	Middle energizer stage patterns	Inclusions：Middle energizer patterns；Middle burner patterns；Middle region patterns
472	下焦证	Lower energizer stage patterns	Inclusions：Lower burner patterns；Lower region patterns
473	其他特指的三焦证	Other specified triple energizer stage patterns	
474	未特指的三焦证	Triple energizer stage patterns, unspecified	
475	卫气营血证	Four phase patterns	Inclusions：Wenbing Aspect Patterns
476	卫分证	Defense phase patterns	Inclusions：Wei aspect patterns
477	湿遏卫阳证	Dampness obstructing the defense yang pattern	
478	温邪侵袭肺卫证	Heat attacking the lung defense pattern	Inclusions：Warm attacking the lung defense pattern
479	其他特指的卫分证	Other specified defense phase patterns	
480	未特指的卫分证	Defense phase patterns, unspecified	
481	气分证	Qi phase patterns	Inclusions：Qi aspect patterns
482	热入气分证	Heat entering the qi phase pattern	
483	气分湿热证	Qi phase dampness and heat pattern	
484	湿阻气分证	Dampness obstructing the qi phase pattern	
485	其他特指的气分证	Other specified qi phase patterns	
486	未特指的气分证	Qi phase patterns, unspecified	
487	营分证	Nutrient phase patterns	Inclusions：Ying aspect patterns
488	营卫不和证	Nutrient qi and defense qi disharmony pattern	
489	热入营分证	Heat in the nutrient phase pattern	
490	热入营血证	Heat entering the nutrient and blood phase pattern	

continued

序号	中　文	英　文	Inclusions/Exclusions
491	其他特指的营分证	Other specified nutrient phase patterns	
492	未特指的营分证	Nutrient phase patterns, unspecified	
493	血分证	Blood phase patterns	Inclusions：Xue aspect patterns
494	血分证	Blood phase pattern	Inclusions：Blood and heat pattern；Interior harassing pattern；Excess heat in the blood aspect pattern
495	热入血分证	Heat entering the blood phase pattern	
496	其他特指的血分证	Other specified blood phase patterns	
497	未特指的血分证	Blood phase patterns, unspecified	
498	其他特指的卫气营血证	Other specified four phase patterns	
499	未特指的卫气营血证	Four phase patterns, unspecified	
500	四象医学病证	Four constitution medicine patterns	Inclusions：Sasang Constitution Medicine Patterns
501	太阳人病证	Large yang type patterns	Inclusions：Taeyang Type Constitution Patterns；TY Type Constitution Patterns
502	太阳人外感腰脊病证	Large yang type exterior origin lower back pattern	Inclusions：Taeyang type exterior pattern；TY type exterior pattern；Type I constitution patterns of the exterior
503	太阳人内触小肠病证	Large yang type interior origin small intestine pattern	
504	太阳人表里兼病证	Large yang type exterior interior combined pattern	
505	其他特指的太阳人病证	Other specified large yang type patterns	
506	未特指的太阳人病证	Large yang type patterns, unspecified	
507	少阳人病证	Small yang type patterns	Inclusions：Soyang Type Constitution Patterns；SY Type Constitution Patterns
508	少阳人少阳伤风证	Small yang type lesser yang wind damage pattern	
509	少阳人亡阴证	Small yang type yin depletion pattern	
510	少阳人胸膈热证	Small yang type chest heat congested pattern	
511	少阳人阴虚证	Small yang type yin deficit pattern	
512	少阳人表里兼病证	Small yang type exterior interior combined pattern	
513	其他特指的少阳人病证	Other specified small yang type patterns	
514	未特指的少阳人病证	Small yang type patterns, unspecified	

continued

序号	中　文	英　文	Inclusions/Exclusions
515	太阴人病证	Large yin type patterns	Inclusions：Taeeum Type Constitution Patterns；TE Type Constitution Patterns
516	太阴人背顀表病证	Large yin type supraspinal exterior pattern	
517	太阴人胃脘寒证	Large yin type esophagus cold pattern	
518	太阴人肝热证	Large yin type liver heat pattern	
519	太阴人燥热证	Large yin type dryness heat pattern	
520	太阴人表里兼病证	Large yin type exterior Interior combined pattern	
521	其他特指的太阴人病证	Other specified large yin type patterns	
522	未特指的太阴人病证	Large yin type patterns, unspecified	
523	少阴人病证	Small yin type patterns	Inclusions：Soeum type constitution patterns
524	少阴人郁狂证	Small yin type congestive hyperpsychotic pattern	
525	少阴人亡阳证	Small yin type yang depletion pattern	
526	少阴人太阴证	Small yin type greater yin pattern	
527	少阴人少阴证	Small yin type lesser yin pattern	
528	少阴人表里兼病证	Small yin type exterior interior combined pattern	
529	其他特指的少阴人病证	Other specified small yin type patterns；	
530	未特指的少阴人病证	Small yin type patterns, unspecified	
531	其他特指的四象医学病证	Other specified four constitution medicine patterns	
532	未特指的四象医学病证	Four constitution medicine patterns, unspecified	
533	其他特指的传统医学证候	Other specified traditional medicine patterns	
534	未特指的传统医学证候	Traditional medicine patterns, unspecified	
535	其他特指的传统医学病证-模块1	Other specified supplementary Chapter Traditional Medicine Conditions — Module I	
536	未特指的传统医学病证-模块1	Supplementary Chapter Traditional Medicine Conditions — Module I, unspecified	

（英文版来源于世界卫生组织 2018 年 6 月 18 日发布的 ICD-11 传统医学章节，中文版来源于国家卫生健康委编译的 ICD-11 中文版）